# Ninjutsu Safeguards

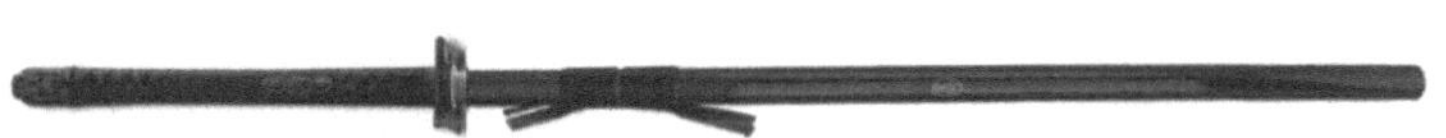

## Strategies in a Time of Quarantine

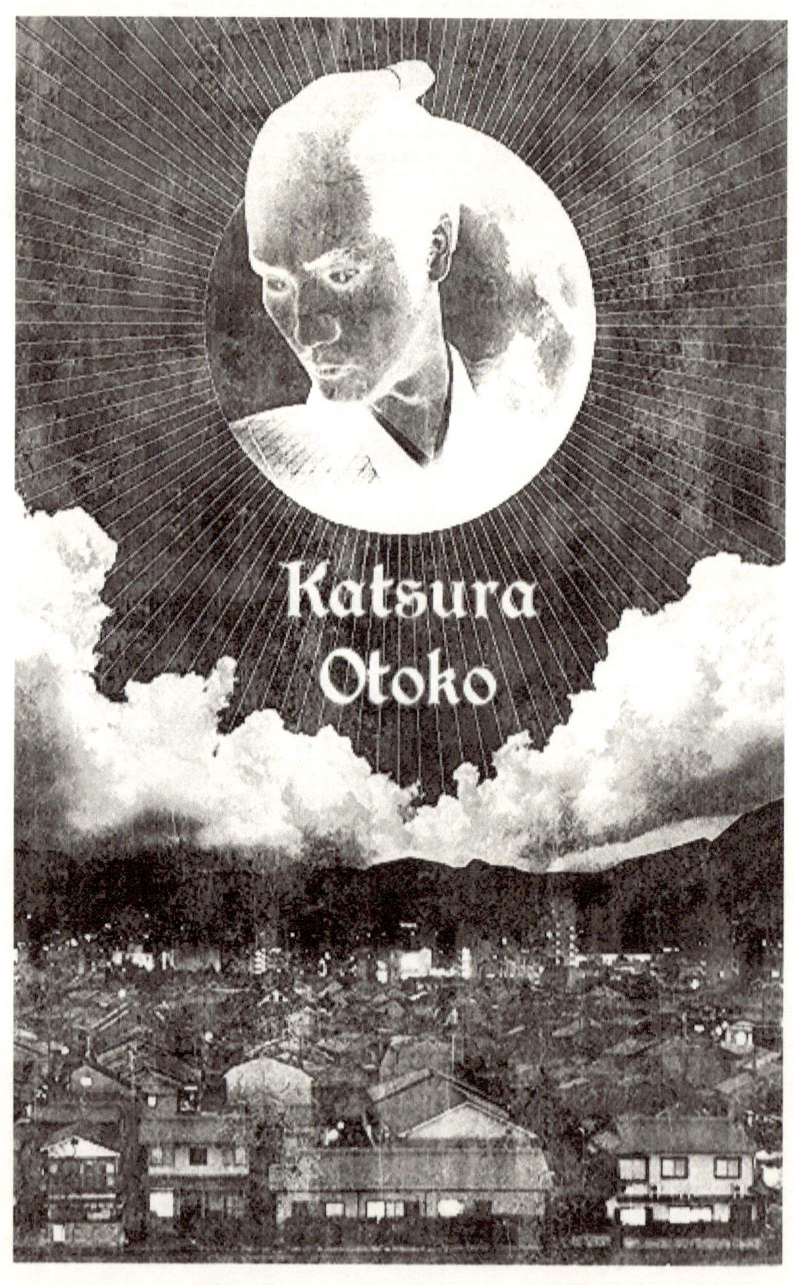



*Katsura Otoko*—alone, without support, as if you are the *Man on the Moon*

# NINJUTSU SAFEGUARDS

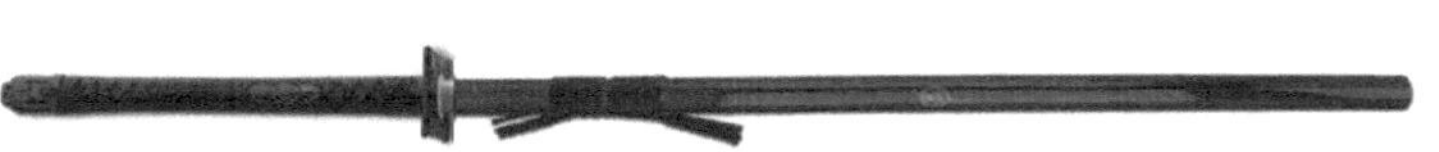

## Strategies in a Time of Quarantine

Volume II in the *Katsura Otoko* Series

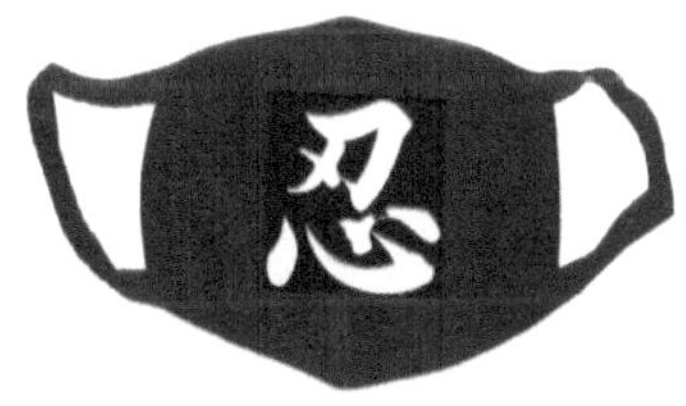

### JAMES LORIEGA

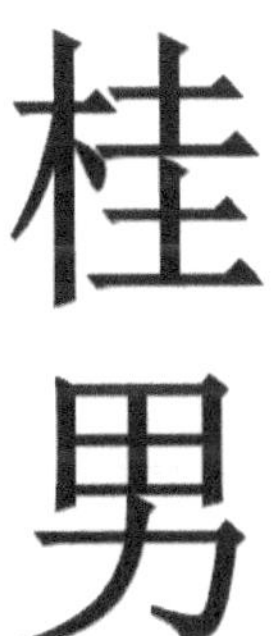

LOST ARTS
PUBLICATIONS

Book design by Junzo Hirose
Art and graphics by Rodolfo Sarmiento
Jacket design by Jason Handsome

NINJUTSU SAFEGUARDS: Strategies in a Time of Quarantine
Volume II of the *Katsura Otoko* series


Second Printing: April 2021

ISBN: 978-1-716-10752-8

Lost Arts Publications
Brooklyn, NY 11235

**LOST ARTS
PUBLICATIONS**

**Limit of Liability / Disclaimer of Warranty**

The information presented in this book is not intended to be interpreted as medical or legal advice; nor is the description of the techniques meant to take the place of proper instruction under the tutelage and supervision of a qualified and competent instructor. The advice and strategies contained herein may not be suitable for your situation. You should consult with a professional where appropriate.

While the publisher and the author have used their best efforts in preparing this book, they make no representations or warranties with respect to the accuracy of completeness of the contents of this book and neither the publisher nor the author shall be liable for any loss of profit or any other commercial damages, including but not limited to special, incidental, consequential, or other life-or-death situations.

Lost Arts Publications also publishes its books in a variety of electronic formats. Some content that appears in print may not be available in electronic books.

Other titles by this author from
**Lost Arts Publications**

THE PATH OF THE NINJA
UNDERSTANDING NINJUTSU
A LEGACY OF LOST ARTS
SONSHI: *Ninjutsu in The Art of War*
SHINOBI ARUKI: *Walking Methods of the Modern Ninja*
ZANKANJO: *The Code of Shinobi*
NINSOGAKU: *The Art of Face-Reading in Ninjutsu*
KATSURA OTOKO: *Ninja Training for the Lone Practitioner*
LOST WRITINGS OF NINJUTSU

**About the Publisher**

**Lost Arts Publications** is an American book publishing company head-quartered in New York City. Established in 2015 to satisfy interest in unique and almost-lost martial disciplines from both Eastern and Western perspectives, Lost Arts Publications produces niche-focused works on lesser-known and rarely-seen methods.

Two additional imprints also publish under the Lost Arts Publications banner. The *Pay-Per-Cut Press* imprint is dedicated to edged weapons and systems of European origin; while the *Raven Tradecraft Press* imprint specializes in modern spycraft and civilian tradecraft.

Lost Arts Publications are printed in the United States of America
and distributed by Amazon.com and Lulu.com.

# Dedication

---

This volume of the Katsura Otoko series is dedicated to
Ramon Martinez and Jeannette Acosta-Martinez,
Maestri of Bladed Strategies

*Like Katsura Otoko (the Man on the Moon), may you ever
remain steadfast, observant, and self-reliant.*

The **Sonshi** teaches us ...

*Do not to rely on the likelihood of the enemy's not coming,
but on our own readiness to receive him:
not on the chance of his not attacking,
but rather on the fact that we have
made our position unassailable.*

—Sonbu

# Ninjutsu Safeguards

## Strategies in a Time of Quarantine

### Contents

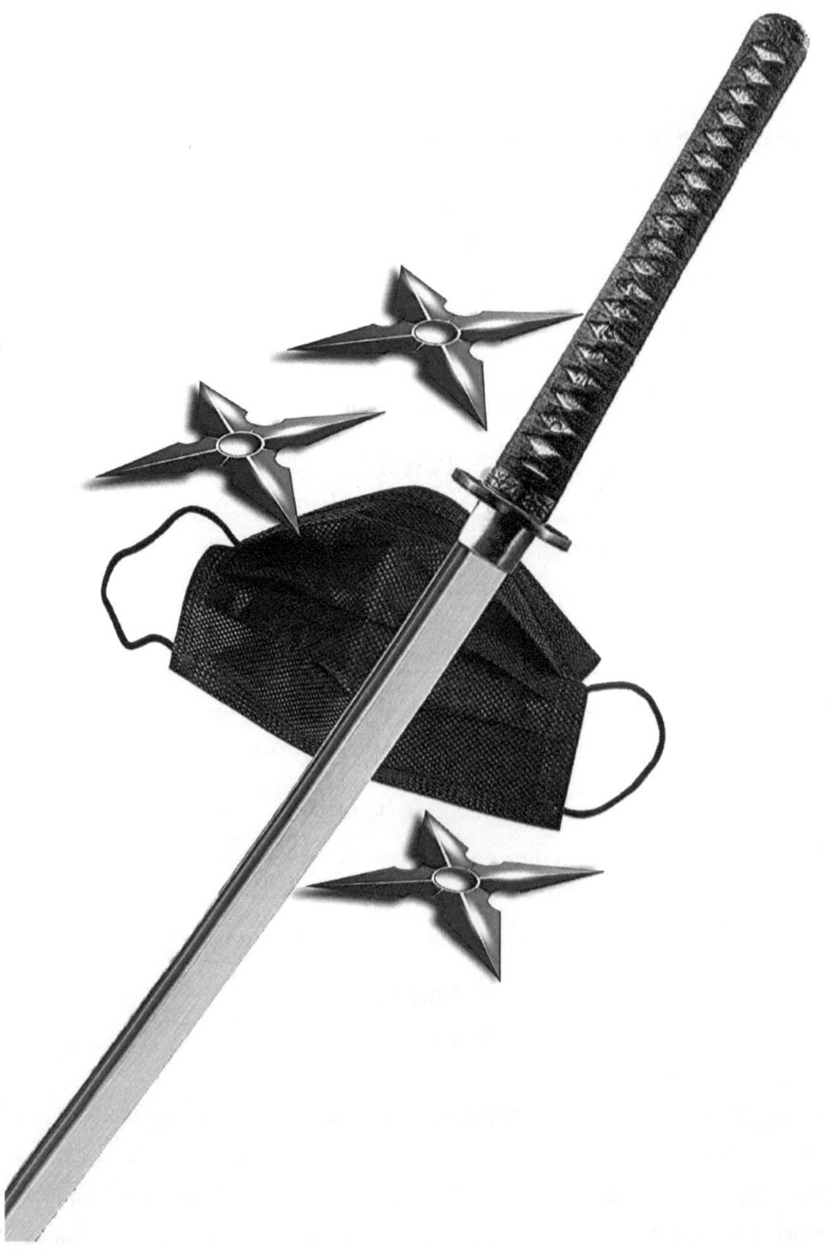

The tragic situation that we—along with the rest of the world—find ourselves in has forced us to make sweeping adjustments to our routine activities and interactions. Safety protocols involving masks, gloves, and proper coughing and sneezing must be practiced; prescribed distances must be adhered to; and rigorous measures of hygiene must be implemented and maintained. Visiting or gathering at restaurants, bars, going to the movies, and attending concerts or sporting events has been curtailed, if not prohibited. And, of course, our dojo, gyms, and fencing salles are off-limits until further notice.

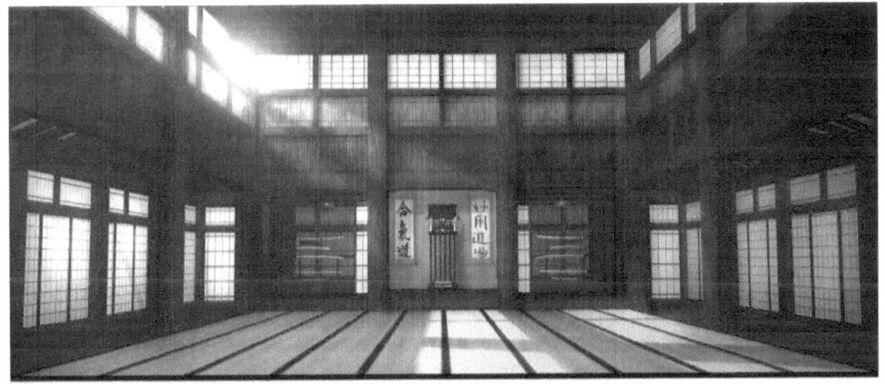

*Dojo*—Off Limits Until Further Notice

Yet while health officials insist that we minimize our contact with others, their rarely-enforced mandates are not uniformly adhered to by many members of the public that we encounter during our inevitable excursions out of doors. Doctors' offices and clinics, pharmacies and drug stores, barber shops and beauty salons, mass transit hubs, supermarkets, public parks, and an inestimable number of necessary venues can be the scene of potentially unhealthy encounters with individual unconcerned with the well-being of others —or even of their own.

As essential personnel, many of us are not afforded the option of avoiding the more defiant scofflaws who are adamant about not having their "freedoms" impinged upon while they blithely impinge on ours. In such cases, our own rigid observance of the mandated protocols or of social distancing may be insufficient.

The irony in all this is that while such individuals can pose serious threats to our health, we, as practitioners of the martial arts, may *not* legally defend ourselves as we might against a lesser, physical danger. We may apply an arm-lock and subdue an assailant who grabs us by the lapels, but we may not respond physically against an unmasked individual who is coughing or sneezing as he approaches us!

In this volume of the *Katsura Otoko* series we present the reader with potential strategies for avoiding and evading such *de facto* assailants who, without raising a fist or a weapon, can render greater harm to us than the armed mugger who demands our wallet ... a wallet we might willingly surrender to avoid receiving a sneeze on our face.

# Part I:
# Core Concepts

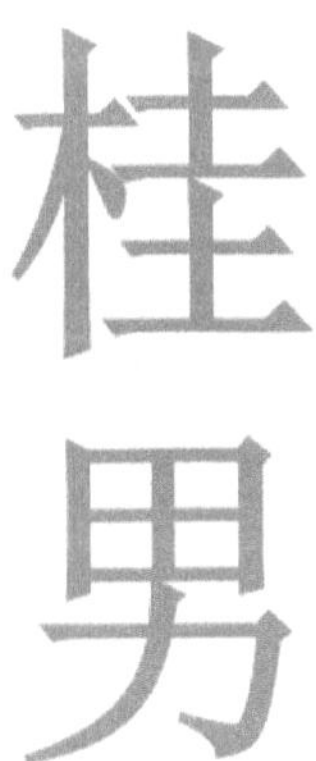

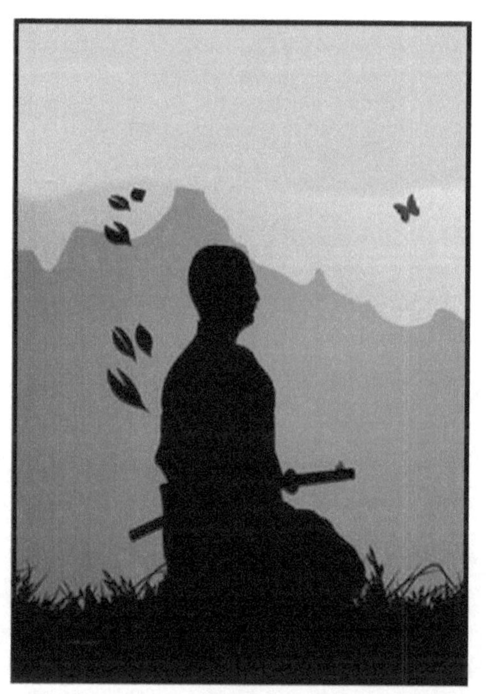

# INTRODUCTION

Martial arts scholar and practitioner Donn F. Draeger once eloquently described **Ninjutsu** as "the Art of Protection Against Danger." For those unfamiliar with this discipline, ninjutsu is not actually a "martial art" in the sense that the term is used today. This is because, in its current sense, the term *martial art* typically refers to a system that focuses on self defense and fighting. Ninjutsu is a system focused principally on intelligence-gathering and espionage. If and when a potential threat is perceived, the ninjutsu practitioner will likely respond to it with one of three strategies: *avoid*, *evade*, or *deceive* the threat.

It is only when the ninjutsu practitioner has failed in those efforts that he/she may resort to the fourth and final strategy—*engage*. It is only for those extreme situations when engagement becomes the final option that ninjutsu teaches the use of armed and unarmed combat methods similar to mainstream martial arts: (martial arts with which ninjutsu is *erroneously* categorized.)

## The Art of Protection Against Danger

Due to its overarching focus of *protecting against danger*, many of ninjutsu's important disciplines can be trained in and developed *without* leaving your desk or your computer. The properly-trained ninjutsu practitioner can gather intelligence, acquire information, anticipate or predict likely attacks (whether of a political, financial, legal, or personal nature), and outwit, deceive, or otherwise thwart a potential adversary—without leaving his desk or assuming a combative posture.

Of course, the ninjutsu practitioner will *still* have to get up from your chair to train and ensure that your body is fit to engage in combat, should that ever become an *unanticipated need,* but the time spent gathering information from his human assets, or reviewing OSINT, SIGINT, IMINT, and other source of intelligence on the computer forms the *core of his ninjutsu.*

### Timeless Advice for Today

One of the foundational influences on the development of Ninjutsu was the military treatise known in the West as **The Art of War**, reputedly written by the strategist, Sun Tzu. That treatise, which in Japan is called the **Sonshi**, contains many admonitions, including—

> *Do not to rely on the likelihood of the enemy's not coming,*
> *but on our own readiness to receive him:*
> *not on the chance of his not attacking,*
> *but rather on the fact that we have*
> *made our position unassailable.*

Today, Sun Tzu's counsel remains as relevant as when it was written 2,500 years. More significantly, it remains relevant not only against the human enemy, which was the threat in Sun Tzu's time, but also against the *invisible and insidious* one—the virus—which threatens in ours. If, as the late Donn Draeger proposed, Ninjutsu *is* the art of protection against danger, then the virus is one of the dangers it can help protect us from.

# THE ESSENCE OF NINJUTSU

### *The Philosophy of the Art*

When you strip away its disciplined movements, its physical skills, its lethal fighting arts, weapons, and equipment, the art of ninjutsu exists as a set of philosophical beliefs and tenets. It is those beliefs and tenets —established to keep its exponents safe from all danger—that shape ninjutsu's strategies. And it is ninjutsu's strategies that shape and determine the methods we practice.

Moreover, the philosophical principles that represent the core of ninjutsu also dictate the ninja's mindset, focus, priorities, and methods. It is these principles that provide the fortitude for remaining constant and consistent in his/her thoughts and actions, particularly when operating alone and without support,

### "Attacks By Infection"

In the first volume of this series, **Ninjutsu Training for the Lone Practitioner**, we defined the theory, mindset, and applications related to *katsura otoko*. This present volume will focus on practices for maintaining your health and well-being in an environment where anyone can be a *de facto* attacker of sorts. It may be an "unintended attack" by an individual who is unaware of his infected tatus; or it may be an "indifferent attack" by one who doesn't guard his health and doesn't care about yours. Whichever the case, we will present ways by which your mind becomes the weapon to defend against such subtle, non-physical, but nonetheless deadly "attacks by infection."

The information in this volume does not depend on exercise equipment or a training partner. In the spirit of *katsura otoko*, training can be undertaken in solitary manner, as would a lone ninja assigned to live behind enemy lines.

## The Essence of Ninjutsu

*is the proactive practice of the strategies, tactics, safeguards, and methods that shield you from danger.*

# THE ESSENCE OF KATSURA OTOKO

In 1959, the renown ninjutsu researcher, Okuse Heishichiro, published a number of ninjutsu tomes, one of which was titled **The Secret Thoughts and Strategies of the Ninja**. In that work Okuse, who in his time was regarded as "the foremost authority on Ninjutsu in Japan," explained that ninja were potentially trained in ten distinct infiltration strategies for "laying the groundwork prior to the outbreak of a military battle." Such groundwork was planned and executed far in advance of the fighting.

## The Term *Katsura Otoko*

The first strategy on Okuse's list is called ***katsura otoko-no-jutsu***, or *the method of the Man on the Moon*. A ninja operating behind enemy lines was referred to as *katsura otoko* since he was almost as isolated as if he were living on the moon. Such an agent, residing and working inside the enemy's territory, must be prepared to function alone and independently *for as long as it takes* to accomplish his mission.

## *Katsura Otoko*—a Metaphor for Self-Reliance

Historically, such assignments required the ninja to function as an agent-in-place and serve for months, or even years, without the benefit of assistance or support from other members of his clan. In that sense, the term *katsura otoko* becomes an apt metaphor for the ninjutsu practitioner today who is cut off, separated, or quarantined, both from members of his dojo and from the outside world. That is to say, you can view the current state of isolation as being similar to the ninja of feudal times, stranded and alone within a hostile environment.

In line with that perspective, the material on these pages can also benefit—

- *the reader interested in practicing ninjutsu but lacking affiliation with a dojo; and*
- *the reader who is affiliated with a ninjutsu system but who, for mandated reasons, is unable to attend training.*

Whichever category you find yourself in, approach the information in this volume as if you are currently a *lone ninja*, striving merely to remain safe, sane, secure, and anonymous—a lone ninja who fully understands that maintaining self-sufficiency and safeguarding one's autonomy requires proactive vigilance a well as routine diligence.

### The Essence of Katsura Otoko

is to *live and maintain a healthy existence*

*while living in a hostile environment.*

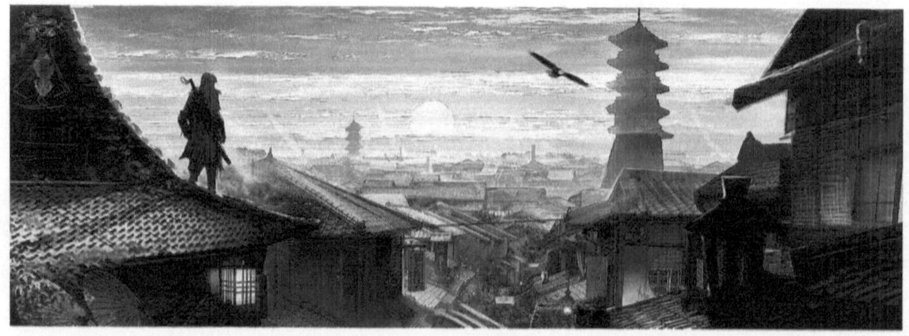

**Maintain a Healthy Existence living in a Hostile  Environment**

# THE ESSENCE OF SELF-RELIANCE



Inherent in the definition of a *warrior* is "one on whom certain people —or certain principles—rely for their existence." Soldiers, for example, go to war because the *people* of their nation rely on them; likewise, a lone individual goes to war—whether a personal one or otherwise— because the principles he believes in *rely* on his upholding them. But while people and principles rely on the warrior to defend them, the warrior can only rely on himself. By necessity, therefore, a warrior must be *self-reliant*.

## Warrior Codes and Creeds

To foster and guide this necessary self-reliance, the warrior develops and adheres to codes and creeds that define his mindset. What follow are two such creeds developed in ages past to inspire self-reliance and provide conviction to those who follow the warrior's paths.

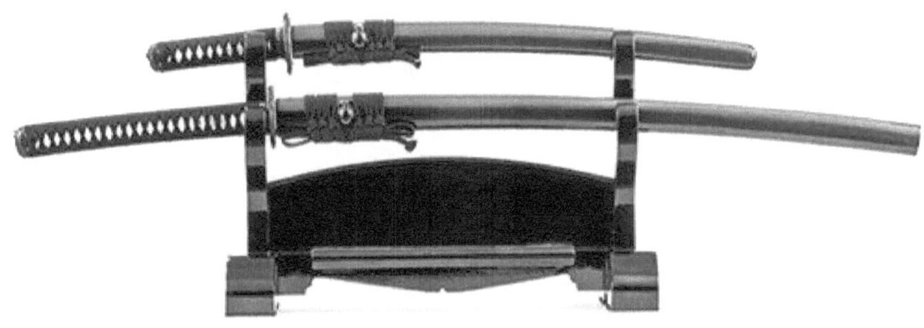

**Unlike the *katana*, the lone shinobi has no companion**

## The Samurai Creed

The twenty-two Zen assertions known as **The Samurai Creed** were reputedly written in the 13th century. These dicta have been ascribed to the strategist, Yamamoto Kansuke, the spymaster for Takeda Shingen, as well as to the master swordsman, Musashi Miyamoto. However, Kansuke died in 1561, and Musashi in 1645 so the Creed origins predates the life of both men.

The earliest English-language translation of The Samurai Creed appears in E.J. Harrison's **The Fighting Spirit of Japan**, first published around 1912. The Creed became more widely-known in the late 1960s with the publication of Charles Gruzanski's, **Spike and Chain**, a 1960s book that focused on two lesser-known weapon arts practiced by the *bushi* and *shinobi*.

Since that time, the Creed has been oft-quoted (and often-mis-interpreted) by martial arts writers from all fighting disciplines. Yet, despite its uncertain provenance and its many imprecise "interpretations," the Creed represents an invaluable resource for aspiring and active ninjutsu practitioners seeking to align their training and their lives with an austere but authentic *Path of the Warrior*, to use a trite expression. For the rare reader who has not yet seen it, The Samurai Creed follows in its most original form. Interpret it as you will for, given the current situation, each student must become his own teacher.

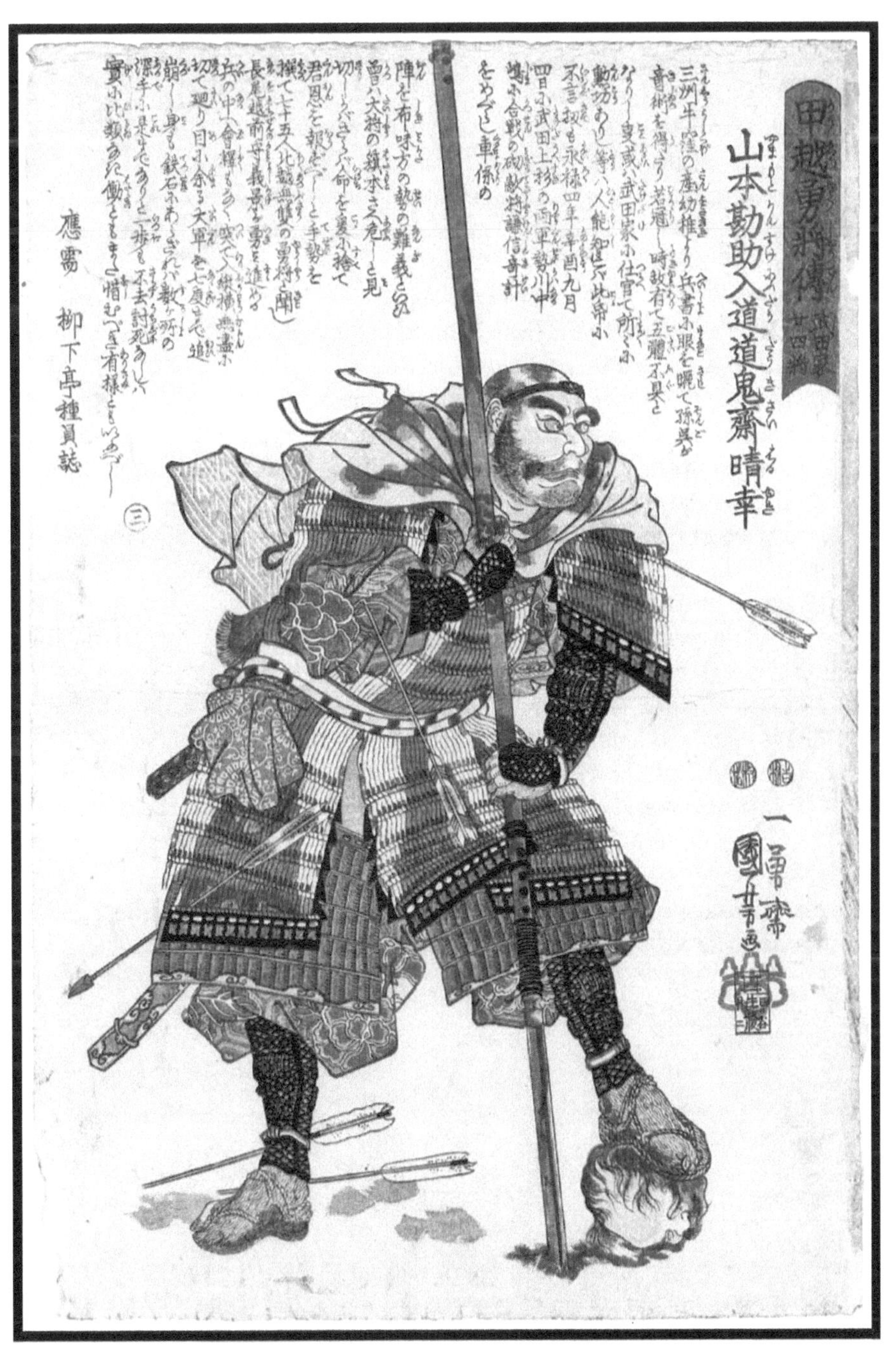

Yamamoto Kansuke, as popularly depicted

# The Samurai Creed

*I have no parents; I make the heavens and the earth my parents.*

*I have no home; I make* **seika tanden**[1] *(abdominal region) my home.*

*I have no divine power; I make honesty my divine power.*

*I have no means; I make docility my means.*

*I have no magic power; I make personality my magic power.*

*I have neither life nor death; I make of* **a um** (the art of regulating one's breath) *my life and death.*

*I have no body; I make stoicism my body.*

*I have no eyes; I make the flash of lightning my eyes.*

*I have no ears; I make sensibility my ears.*

*I have no limbs; I make promptitude my limbs.*

*I have no laws; I make self-protection my laws.*

*I have no strategy; I make* **sakkatsu jizai**[2] (free to kill and free to restore life) *my strategy.*

*I have no designs; I make* **kisan** (seizing opportunity by the forelock) *my designs.*

*I have no miracles; I make righteous laws my miracle.*

*I have no principles; I make* **rinkiohen** (adaptability to all of life's circumstances) *my principle.*

*I have no tactics; I make* **kyo-jitsu** (emptiness and fullness) *my tactics.*

*I have no talent; I make* **toi sokumyo**[3] (ready wit) *my talent.*

*I have no friends; I make my mind my friend.*

*I have no enemies; I make  a lack of caution my enemy.*

*I have no armor; I make* **jin-gi**[4] (benevolence and righteousness[5]) *my armor.*

*I have no castle; I make* **fudoshin** (immovable mind) *my castle.*

*I have no sword; I make* **mushin** (absence of self) *my sword.*

---

1 Another term for the *hara*.

2 This is similar to the samurai privilege of *Kirisute Gomen*, the warrior's right to kill and walk away.

3 This is the attribute of *resourcefulness* that is so critical for spies and covert agents.

4 These virtues are taken directly from *Bushido*, the code of conduct of the Bushi.

5 Benevolence and righteousness are two of the Virtues in the Code of Bushido.

## The Dokkōdō

Although, as has been indicated, Musashi Miyamoto did not write The Samurai Creed, he did in fact author a number of significant writings that are still timely today. The first, of course, is his classic **Go Rin-no-Sho**, or *Book of Five Rings*, Musashi's venerated tome on strategy written under the guise of a sword manual. It is, however, his lesser-known advice on living that interests us here.

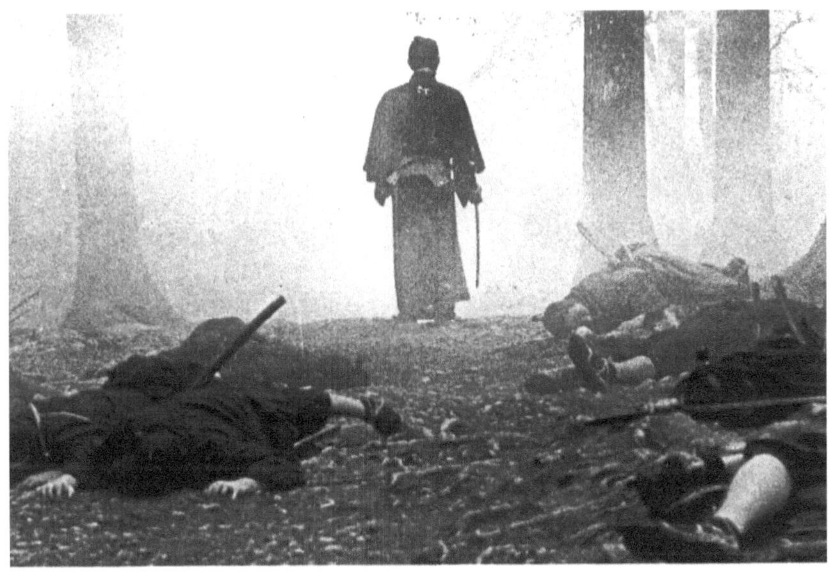

The **Dokkōdō**, a term variously translated as *The Way Alone, The Way to Go Forth Alone*, or *The Way of Walking Alone*, is a short work written by Musashi the week before he died in 1645. Its list of twenty-one precepts was written as a final letter to his favorite disciple, Terao Magonojō. The precepts represent the sword master's counsel on how to live a stringent but righteous and honest life. Anyone who chooses to walk alone—free from societal influences—will discover great value in them.

25

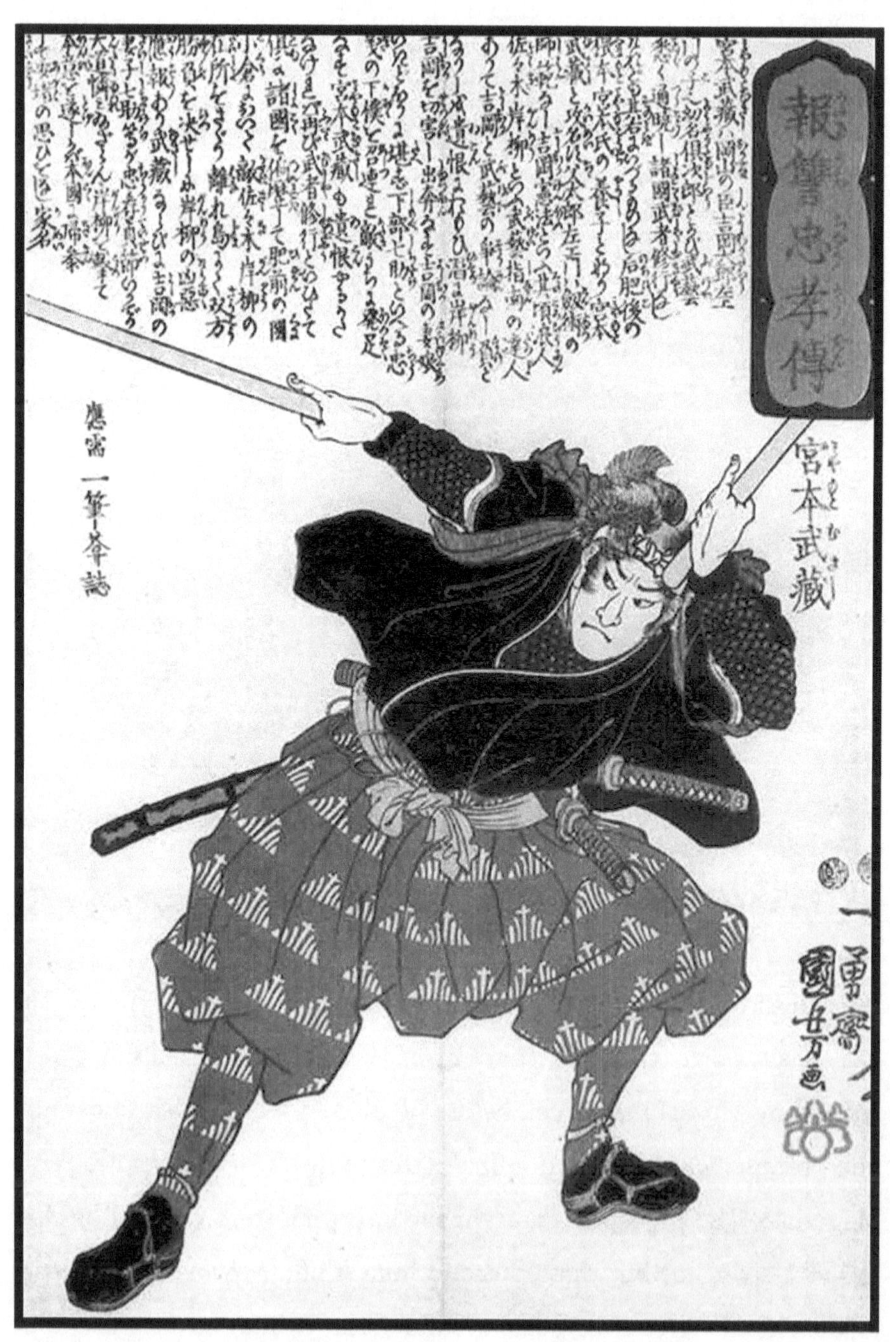

Musashi Miyamoto, as popularly depicted

# The Way Alone

1. *Accept everything just the way it is.*
2. *Do not seek pleasure for its own sake.*
3. *Do not give preference to anything among all things.*
4. *Think lightly of yourself and deeply of the world.*
5. *Be detached from desire your whole life.*
6. *Do not regret what you have done.*
7. *Never be jealous.*
8. *Never let yourself be saddened by a separation.*
9. *Resentment and complaint are appropriate neither for oneself nor others.*
10. *Do not let yourself be guided by the feeling of lust or love.*
11. *Do not seek elegance and beauty in all things.*
12. *Be indifferent to where you live.*
13. *Do not pursue the taste of good food.*
14. *Do not hold on to possessions you no longer need.*
15. *Do not act following customary beliefs.*
16. *Do not collect weapons or practice with weapons beyond what is useful.*
17. *Do not fear death.*
18. *Do not seek to possess either goods or fiefs for your old age.*
19. *Respect Buddha and the gods without counting on their help.*
20. *You may abandon your own body but you must preserve your honor.*
21. *Never depart from the Way[6] [of the Martial Arts.]*

Whether one follows the *Samurai Creed* of anonymous provenance, the *Dokkodo* of Musashi Miyamoto—or some other relevant set of tenets—it should be one that bolsters body, mind, and spirit as an integrated whole. Integrity, as will be seen in the next section, is fundamentally what keeps us comporting ourselves in full alignment with our goals and objectives.

---

6 Musashi's use of the term *Way* refers as much to the concept of the *Tao*, as to the concept of *michi*, or "life path."

**The Essence of Self Reliance is**

the *ability to think, decide, and do for yourself in the absence of*

*allies, equipment, or resources.*

# Part II:

# TRADITIONAL TEACHINGS

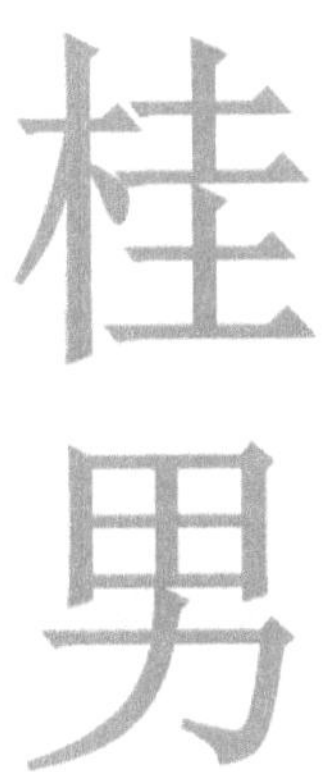

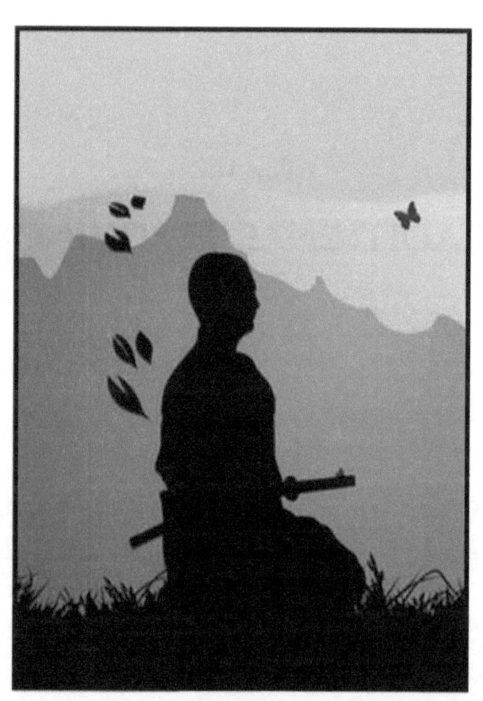

# THE MIND AS A WEAPON

Ninjutsu is an art first practiced in the mind, and it is a person's mindset that makes them a ninja. As ninjutsu practitioners, we are more fortunate than martial artists because the art we practice encompasses a vast number of philosophical, psychological, and physical teachings that serve to guide our thinking and inform our *actions*.

Tthe ninja was paid to do what the samurai could not. While the samurai was paid to fight, the ninja was paid not to outfight the enemy but to *outsmart* him. For that reason, the ninja's profession mandated that he use his *mental* weapons before he resorted to physical ones.

## Shinrigaku

Although in modern Japanese usage the term *shinrigaku* is used to mean "psychology," it was originally used as blanket term for the variety of *mental strategies* used by the ninja against an enemy or opponent. The term encompassed covert methods of character assessment, face-reading, hypnotism, persuasion, elicitation (a form of covert interrogation), manipulation, and related skills.

In **The Secret Thoughts and Strategies of the Ninja**, mentioned in Part I, Heishichiro Okuse observes that ninja regarded nothing as impossible[7] and scientifically applied what he calls "brain power" to

---

7 In the third film of the 1960s *Shinobi-no-Mono* series, Ishikawa Goemon tells Hattori Hanzo, "*The greatest shame for a shinobi is to assume any objective is*

every problem they encountered. He further identified the non-physical aspects of ninjutsu as being the key to a successful career as a shinobi.

In **Ninja, The Invisible Assassin**s, Adams notes,

> [The ninja] *had to have their wits about them at all times and* [to] *work out complicated problems on the spot. They learned to sharpen their perception and insight, developing their instincts to a point that seemed almost superhuman.*

That methodical *"sharpening of perception and insight"*, and *"development of instincts to a point that seemed almost superhu*man" is what is known in ninjutsu as *shinrigaku*. Regrettably, it is taught in merely a handful of modern ninjutsu dojo.

## Mind Disciplines

Mind disciplines evolved over time in feudal Japan, when the potential for life-or-death engagements was present at all times. The disciplines warned the bushi and shinobi if danger was imminent, allowing them to preempt the threat. More importantly, by the early insight they provided, these disciplines enabled the bushi to avert unnecessary fighting.

Shinrigaku served the shinobi as it did the bushi, but for a different reason. The shinobi had to avoid open combat for purposes of anonymity and the integrity of their assignments. Unless they planned to leave a trail of dead or injured bodies that would lead to their being

---

*impossible."*
32

discovered, the shinobi had to rely on disciplines that alerted them to potential danger and precluded the need for combat or killing.

## Koryū Bugei and Gendai Budo

At this point we must understand the difference between fighting arts and martial arts within the context of historical Japanese combat disciplines. Actual fighting arts actively used prior to 1868 are designated as **koryū bugei**, or technically "old school arts (crafts) of war." These include jujutsu, kenjutsu, ninjutsu, and other disciplines used in battle. Systems that were developed after 1868 are designated as **gendai budo**, or "modern martial ways." They include judo, kendo, karate, aikido; though they are called "martial arts," they were never used in battle and are actually *arts for self-defense*.

Traditionally, *shinrigaku* disciplines were acquired by the bushi and shinobi in the practice of their *koryū bugei* arts. Today, they have been virtually lost in the wake of the *gendai budo*. This is because once the possibility of someone lying in wait with sharp *katana* is no longer a likely threat and the skills that once evolved for averting such once-prevalent threats have waned or died. The chapters that immediately follow will each address distinct components of *shinrigaku*.

The tenets that follow have been taught in ninjutsu for centuries. I chose them from among countless others as examples of how ninjutsu's teachings are perennial and relevant to the current pandemic situation. By keeping the tenets in mind we can use them to re-frame our present perspective.

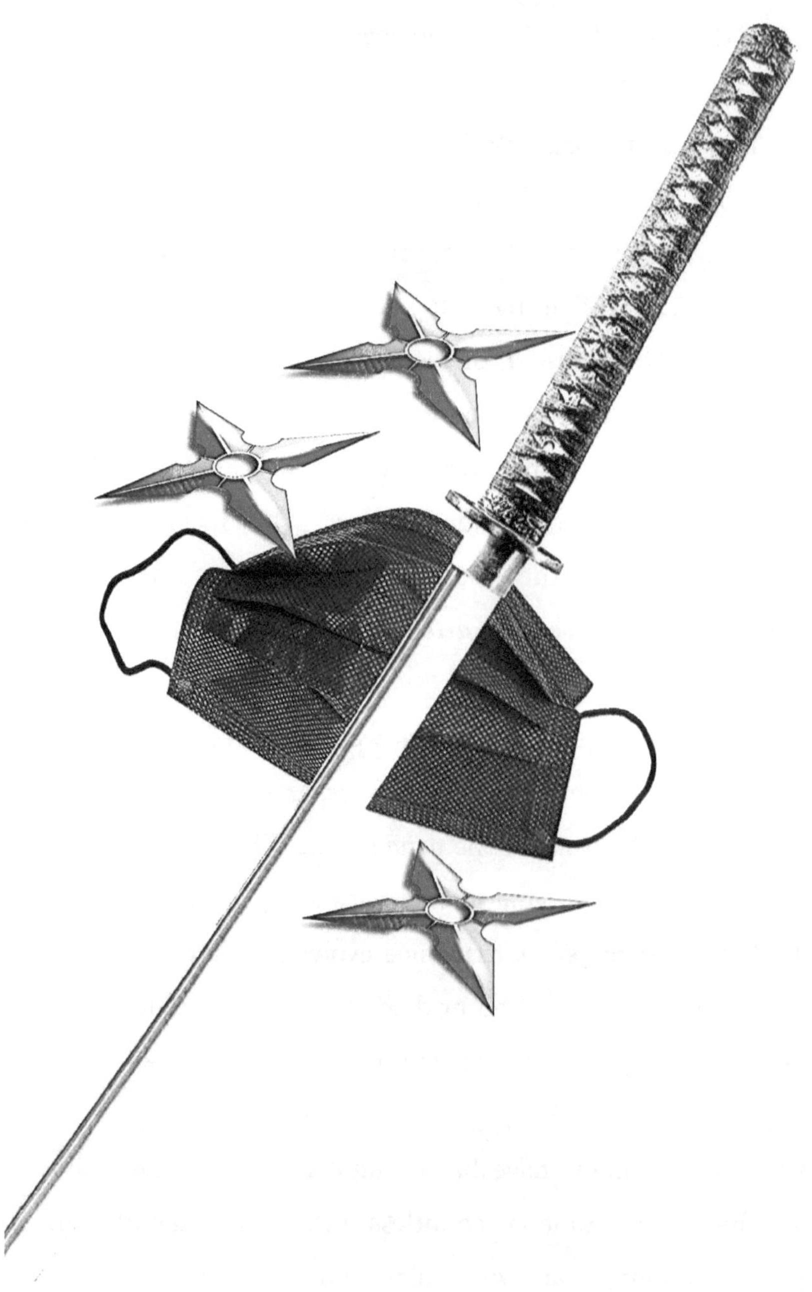

# METSUKE

*If your mind is preoccupied with one leaf, you will not see the others; if you don't focus your attention on one, you will see hundreds and thousands of leaves.*

—Yagyu Munenori
*The Way of the Living Sword*

**Metsuke**, like most Japanese words, carries multiple meanings in the *koryū* arts. Literally "ability to see," *metsuke* can be used to describe—1) the way in which you *gaze* at an opponent; 2) the way in which you *view* a dangerous situation; or 3) the manner in which you *regard* a threatening environment. In applying metsuke, you use your eyes perceptively, *without* obsessive focus or undue analysis. Within the context of ninjutsu and the *koryū bugei*, metsuke can be expressed as a *piercing* or *penetrating gaze,* and is an attribute developed through training and experience.

## Your Facial Expression

It is first important to remember that facial expressions and demeanor openly provide information about an individual's state of mind. Knowing that, you must keep your own face *impassive* in combat so that it cannot be easily read by an astute enemy.

Similarly, avoid attempt to intimidate an enemy using facial expressions; a person who makes exaggerated, fearsome, or threatening faces is perceived as insecurity or desperation, like a child trying to frighten an adult. Actively assess and analyze your enemy, but your decisions ad  intentions must not be reflected on you face.

## Mokushin and Ganriki

In the information the follows, we will refer to the metsuke as the *combat gaze*. Although there are many ways to apply the combat gaze, there are two principal ways that relate directly to active combative engagement. The first way is called *mokushin, or* "the eye of the mind;" the second way is *ganriki,* or "the power of the eye."

## Mokushin

*Mokushin* involves seeing with the *mind's eye*, often to enclose and envelope an opponent. This is best accomplished by maintaining a *calm, natural,* and *confident* expression on the face. Projecting a serene demeanor regardless of what happens is much more unsettling to an enemy than an angry war face. A calm face allows you to remain calm, and this in turn helps you to observe and assess the enemy—without wasting energy by attempting to intimidate or deceive him.

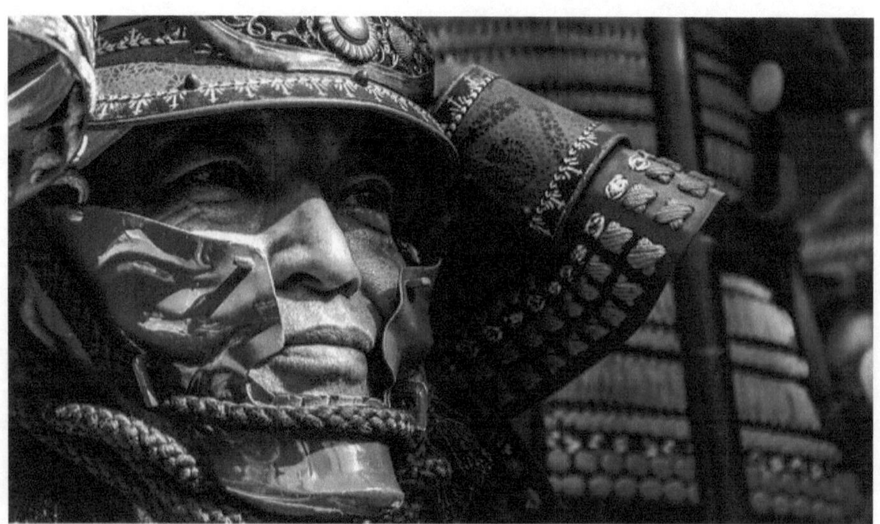

**Mokushin, the Calm, Confident, and Observant Gaze**

## Ganriki

When your are fully intent on defeating your enemy, your calm face will naturally take on a piercing and intense quality called *ganriki*. Ganriki is a *sharp, penetrating gaze* that sees an enemy's intentions and can be used to dominate and control him. Just as importantly, your enemy will understand this look, as well.

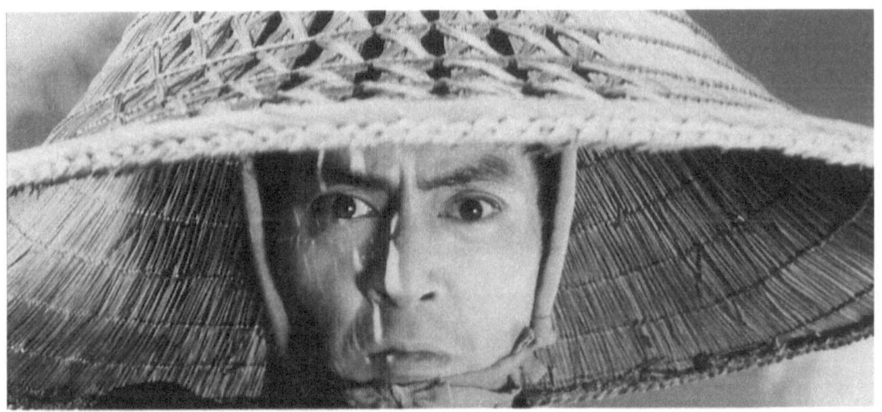

*Ganriki*, the Sharp, Piercing, and Penetrating Gaze

Some traditions teach that one should look directly at the opponent's eyes. Other traditions warn that looking at the eyes can be mesmerizing, and that one should instead look at the whole person from head to toe. Holding your combat gaze just above the bridge of the enemy's nose, between his two eyebrows, is a practical compromise. From there you can also sense intentions from his subtle changes and shifts in posture.

In **The Book of Five Rings** legendary master swordsman, Musashi Miyamoto, eloquently provides the following advice with respect to the *combat gaze* (although Musashi's many translators do not know enough to call it that):

> View situations in a sweeping, broad fashion.
> The two ways of seeing things are **kan** (observing) *and* **ken** (looking). *Kan, observing, is strong; ken, looking, weak. Seeing distant things as if they are close at hand and seeing close things as if they are distant is unique to the art of combat.*

## Pay Attention *Without* Looking

Both unfocused and focused seeing form the spectrum of the combat gaze; but metsuke is not merely unfocused or focused seeing. It requires *paying attention*. Never look into the opponent's eyes because this distracts your clarity of mind. Before he founded **aikido**, *Ueshiba Morihei*, who had trained rigorously in *Daito-ryu* and other *koryū* arts, wrote:

> *Do not look at the opponent's eyes, or your mind will be drawn into them. Do not look at his sword, or you will be slain by it. Do not look at him, or your spirit will be distracted. True budo is the cultivation of attraction with which to draw the whole opponent to you. All I have to do is keep standing this way.*

Thus *mokushin* is used to gaze beyond the enemy, taking in the whole person, noticing every aspect, and thus reading any intention or movement immediately. *Ganriki* is used to control the enemy because it enables you to control the distance between you (*ma-ai*), and thus allows you to appropriately intercept.

## Enzan-no-Metsuke

The phrase *enzan-no-metsuke* translates as, "Gazing at a distant mountain," and represents a common practice used for developing metsuke. It involves focusing the eyes at a distance, which is crucial to developing the mental vision necessary in combat, instead of looking at what is directly in front of you.

To begin *enzan-no-metsuke*, relax your vision and look as if gazing at the panorama behind the training partner. You will begin seeing your surroundings in proper perspective, without locking your focus on a particular detail—which can prevent you from seeing everything else.

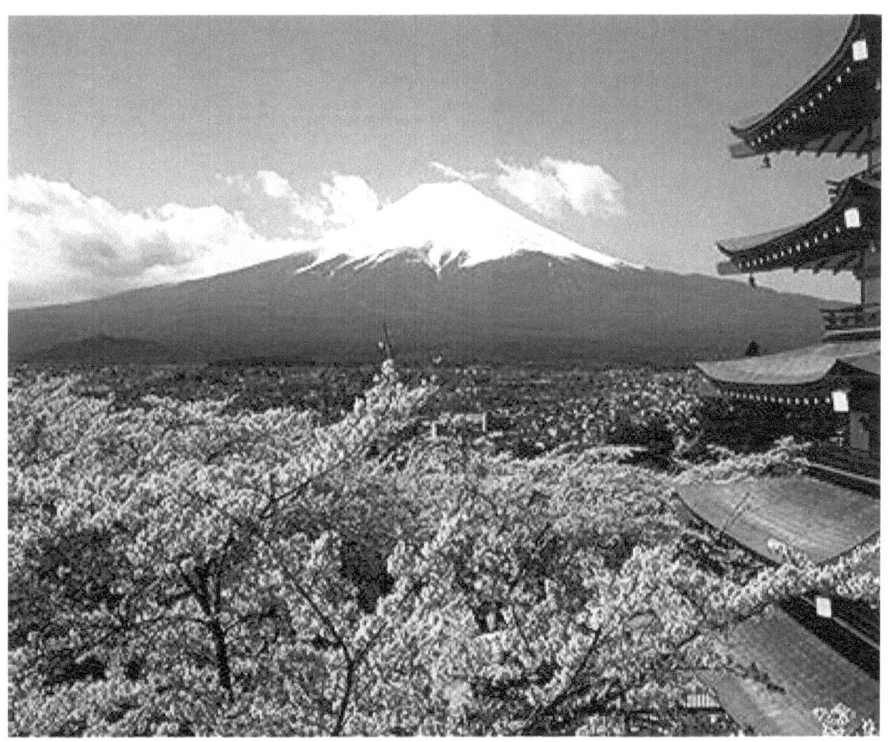

*Enzan-no-Metsuke*, **Gazing at a Distant Mountain** (Fujiyama)

## What You Don't Use ...

Any disregard for using the combat gaze not only robs you of its advantages in a personal combat engagement, but can also atrophy of these faculties. In our "civilized" world we are taught only to look, and thereby we become blind to the threats we should notice. Believing that it is enough to *look*, we cease to *observe*.

For the bushi and shinobi, there were ways to look through water, and there were ways to see into fire. Today, there is more to see in our air than city people would want to know exists! Everything on the planet contains dimensions not readily perceivable to the untrained eye. To seen them, train your eyes!

# BANPEN FUGYO

*Ten Thousand Changes; No Surprises*

**Banpen Fugyo** translates roughly as *"Ten Thousand Changes; No Surprises."* This tenet reminds us to never be surprised by any change, no matter how unexpected. This is admittedly a challenging attribute to develop, and novices can begin by never responding to being surprised and never reacting in a visibly surprised manner. Do not become the proverbial "deer in the headlights."

A shinobi maintains his mental equilibrium regardless of how off-balance he may actually feel, and never allows whatever has caught him off guard to alter his outward demeanor. He may thus experience *ten thousand changes,* but will outwardly demonstrate *no surprise.*

*Banpen fugyo* will serve you in keeping your wits about you during what may feel like uncertain times—*uncertain times such as these.* You must maintain a positive perspective, remembering that nothing good comes from panicking. Turn your legitimate concern into a catalyst for exercising extreme caution in all you do. Engage in constructive "What if" thinking and help those around you to do likewise.

Adopt and embrace an attitude of **fudoshin**. This term is comprised of *fudo,* or "immovable," and *shin,* which means "heart," or "mind," or both. Possessing an attitude of fudoshin means you cannot be made to feel ruffled or frazzled. Possessing fudoshin means that, regardless of what distress you may feel, you remain in control and unperturbed.

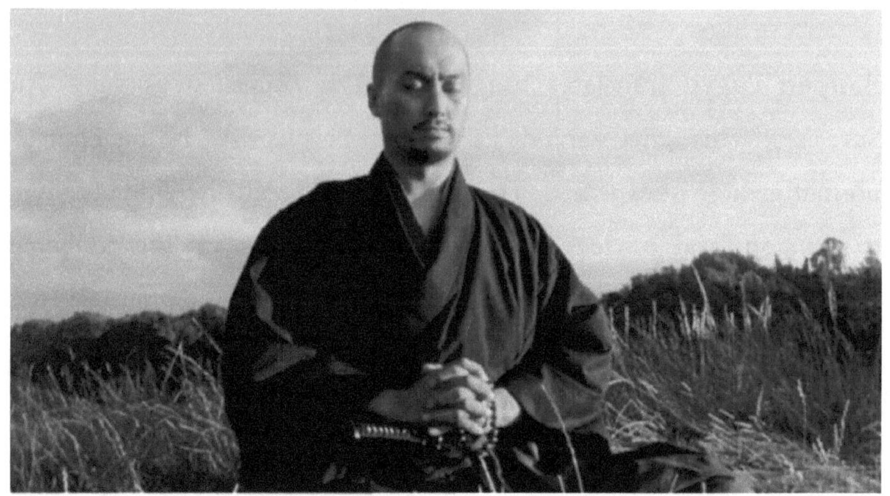

**Fudoshin—in control and unperturbed**

Possessing fudoshin facilitates banpen fugyo, and practicing banpen fugyo enhances fudoshin. You may know fear, but you will never panic! And you may experience ten thousand changes, but within you they will *evoke no change.*

# HARAGEI



—Sonbu
*Sonshi, Book III*

The above quote may sound trite today, but during Japan's bloody *Warring States Era* (1467—1601) it was considered sage military advice. The advice is actually twofold: 1) to *know your enemy*, and 2) to *know yourself*. You begin with the obvious and familiar, *knowing yourself*; and by extension, *developing* yourself. The core attribute on which the ninja's abilities to know his enemy and himself rely is *haragei*.

The following anecdote concerning *Yagyu Munenori*, who was the personal sword instructor to Shogun Iemitsu, is an excellent example of haragei. Writer Makoto Sugawara recounts it as follows:

> *When Munenori was granted an audience with the shogun, Iemitsu, he sat down, put his hands on the tatami floor, as retainers always did to show their respect to their master.*
>
> *Suddenly, Iemitsu thrust a spear at the "unsuspecting" Munenori—and was surprised to find himself lying flat on his back!*
>
> *Munenori had sensed the shogun's intention before a move had been made, and swept Iemitsu's legs out from under him at the instant of the thrust.*

What alerted Munenori to the shogun's failed surprise attack was his keenly-developed sense of *haragei*.

## Haragei

In the *koryū bugei*, haragei refers to a sense or quality that enables the *bushi* and *shinobi* to anticipate danger or perceive an opponent's intentions. Additionally, in a non-combative context haragei can refer to a highly-tuned intuition that allows a person to grasp the true nature of a situation independently of verbal communication or deductive reasoning. A person with haragei will be able to see behind what another person says to what they really mean—and will also be able to successfully hide his own true intentions, if and when necessary.

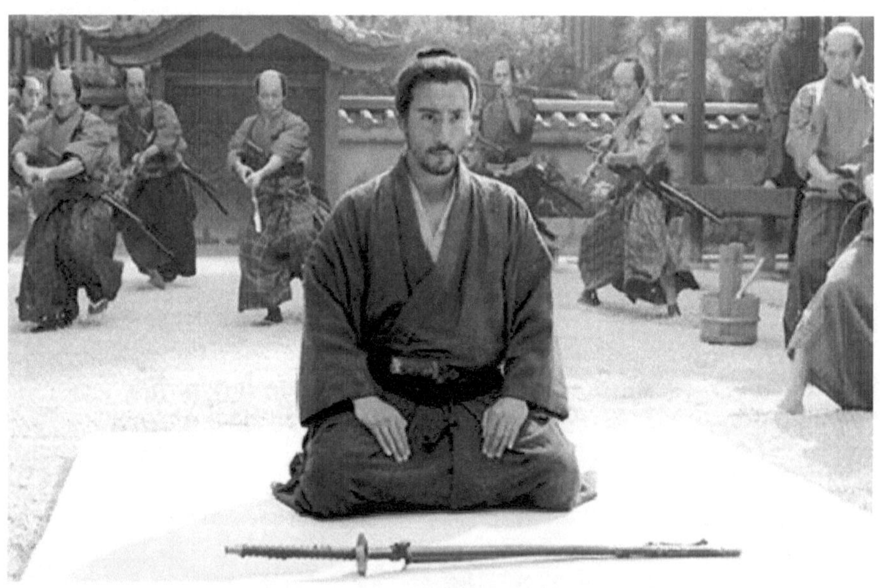

**The ability to sense threats and danger**

It is easy to see how this applies to *koryū* arts, since the process of a conflict usually involves *hiding your own true intent while discovering the intentions of the enemy*; and of using that information to devise various stratagems to defeat him. This, in fact, is how the ninja traditionally operated—but it can only be accomplished when one has developed the haragei needed to sense an enemy's true motives. On the physical level, this is *accomplished* by learning to remain *calm* and *unruffled*[8], thereby allowing the enemy's intent to become clear.

The term haragei is derived from the words *hara*, or "stomach," and *gei*, which is an "art" or "craft." We have all experienced the feeling that we *know* information about an individual or situations in advance, which we may regard as a *hunch* or a *gut feeling*. We do not arrive at such conclusions by means of logic or detailed analysis; instead, these insights often come as a flash of information or a sense of impending danger. It is this heightened form of intuition that the samurai and ninja knew it as haragei.

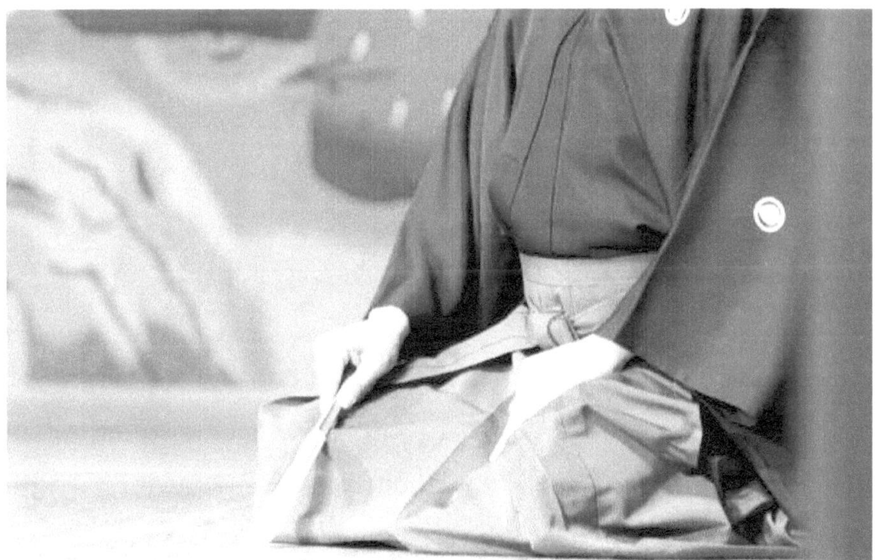

Haragei enables the *shinobi* to sense threats and read intentions

---

8 Expressed as *hara ga suwatte iru*

## Developing Your Haragei

In our fast-paced world there is simply not enough time to digest all the information that is available. Decisions have to be made quickly. Research tells us that 50% of decisions made logically are later proven to be wrong. This is why people taking written exams are often advised to adhere to their first (gut) responses or answers, and to disregard any subsequent impulse to second-guess or change them.

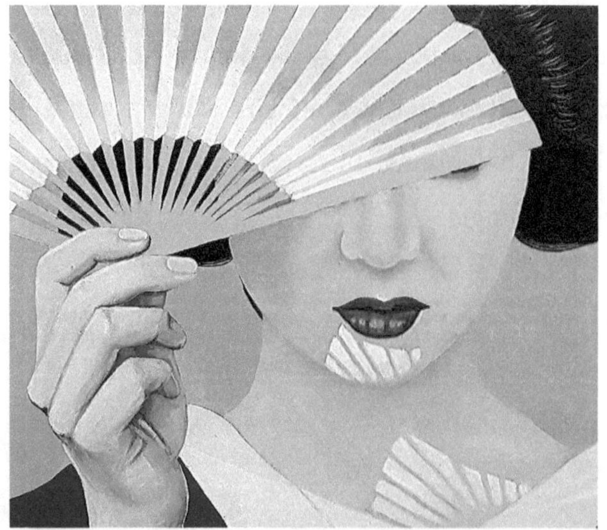

**Discover your enemy's intentions while concealing your own**

Haragei can be developed and accessed intentionally, but only if you train and nurture it. There are many formal methods used for this, as well as some informal modern methods. The best-known method is used in many *koryū* arts and involves formalized breathing exercises that can be practiced at home or in the dojo. One of these is descibed in detail in Section IV, **Staying Honed**.

# SHINSHIN SHINGAN

*The Mind and Eyes of God*

Shinshin Shingan is a shinobi expression that reminds us to enter all situations, whether new or familiar, with *the mind and the eyes of God.* It has been inadequately compared to the overused term "situational awareness," but magnified a hundredfold. As such, it is perhaps one of the most vital principles to espouse at this time.

Although precious little specifics have been written on this subject in the historical ninja manuals still available today, there are relevant words of advice written by Allen W. Dulles, the spymaster who served as Chief of Station for the OSS during WWII, and later became the sixth, and longest-serving, director of the CIA.

Among the **Seventy-Three Rules for Spies** that he set down for his field operatives, Dulles wrote—

- The greatest vice in the Game[9] is that of carelessness. Mistakes made generally cannot be rectified.

- Security consists not only in avoiding big risks. It consists in carrying out daily tasks with painstaking remembrance of the tiny things that security demands. The little things are in many ways more important than the big ones. It is they which oftenest give the Game away. It is consistent care in them which form the habit and characteristic of security mindedness.

---

9 The profession of espionage is referred to as *The Great Game* by those who practice it.

- In any case, the man or woman who does not indulge in the daily security routine, boring and useless though it may sometimes appear, will be found lacking in the proper instinctive reaction when dealing with the bigger issues.

- There are many virtues to be striven after in the job. The greatest of them all is security. All else must be subordinated to that.

Remarkably, these and others of Dulles' *Seventy-Three Rules for Spies* are as applicable today as safeguards against the virus as they were in the 1960s as security protocols for American agents operating in Moscow. In whatever way you accomplish it, the ultimate goal of security-mindedness is to keep yourself safe. It is the same goal you strive for when attempting to develop the *Mind and the Eyes of God.*

While it once served the ninja to foresee a surprise attack from a hidden enemy or a trap at a meeting with a treacherous friend, today *shinshin shingan* must function to keep you healthy and safe from exposure. As Dulles would have agreed, carelessness and a lax attitude are the doors by which a threat enters.

# Part III

# Modern Correlations

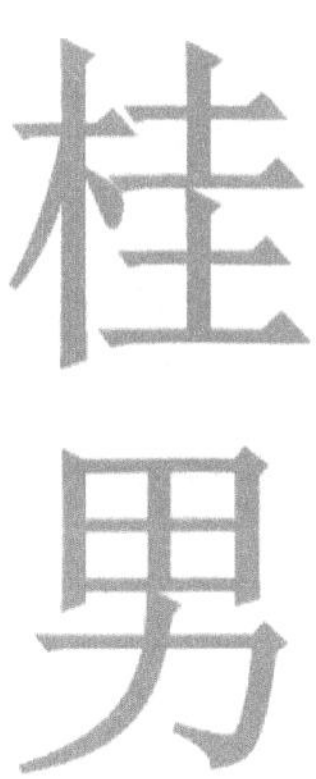

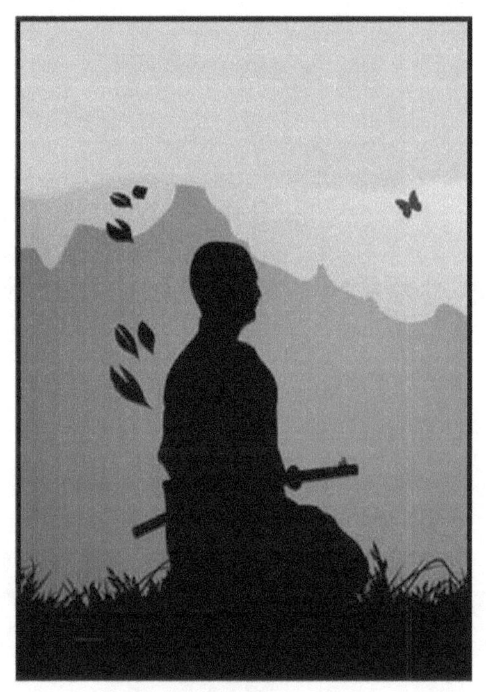

# SENSING DANGER

*An Alternative to Banpen Fugyo*

One of the most advanced teachings of Ninjutsu is *Banpen Fugyo*, addressed in a previous chapter. Translated as having *"Ten Thousand Changes, No Surprises,"* it is an attribute that can be developed and constantly maintained. One way we can begin to develop this attribute at a very rudimentary level by practicing the *Cooper Color Codes*.

## The Cooper Color Codes

The Cooper Color Codes were devised by the late Col. Jeff Cooper's and have been embraced and taught by competent instructors for many decades. In the aftermath of 9/11, the Department of Homeland Security appropriated Cooper's Color Codes and renamed them *Terrorism Alertness Levels* and/or *Terror Threat Levels*. Most people are quite familiar with the concepts, but a review will help to clarify them.

Cooper classified *awareness levels* into four colors that correspond to escalating degrees of preparation for personal protection responses. The system is a mental process, not a physical one, and should be utilized whether or not you are armed. Being aware of the potential for threat that exists at any given time will help you to avoid a deadly threat in the first place, which is always preferable to resorting to a defensive or combative response.

**Condition White**

In condition White, you are relaxed and unaware of what is going on around you. Ideally, a police officer, military person, or citizen should only in White when asleep. Realistically, however, we often drop our guard when we are at home or in some other environment we assume to be safe, like an office or a theater. Yet even police stations have been attacked, so it is better to be more alert whenever you are not at home. If you are attacked in condition White, you may very well die—unless you are lucky. *Luck is not a ninjutsu strategy!*

**Condition Yellow**

In condition Yellow, you remain relaxed, but are aware of who and what is around you. This merely means that you are paying attention to the sights and sounds that surround you whether you are at home or moving in society. Condition Yellow does not equate with paranoia or any other irrational fear of persons or places. Instead, you have simply raised your awareness to a level of attention that will prevent you from being totally surprised by a quickly-changing situation or the unexpected actions of another person.

While walking through *any* area you will loosely keep track of anyone behind you. When choosing a seat in a restaurant, you will position yourself to see the entrance or minimize the number of people seated behind you. You don't need to insist on sitting with your back to a dead corner and your face to the entrance, because you are not anticipating a threat—you are merely conducting an inventory of your surroundings and the people around you.

You will also run through a cursory "what if" visualization of where a threat could appear and what your response should be. If you are attacked in condition Yellow, it should not come as a total surprise. Your response to a threat should have been pre-planned to some extent, allowing you to simply initiate an existing plan rather than having to quickly make one up. A prepared individual *must* be in condition Yellow whenever they are outside the safety of their home.

**Condition Orange**

In condition Orange, you have identified something of interest that may or may not prove to be a threat. Until you determine the true nature of whatever has piqued your interest, your "radar" is narrowed to concentrate on the potential threat, and will remain so focused until you are satisfied no threat exists. Any contact you make with unfamiliar or unknown individuals throughout your day—either incidental or self-initiated—are obvious examples of a condition Orange focus. You know these people are not currently a threat, or you would move swiftly and smoothly to the next higher color. Instead, these individuals simply *could* be a threat, so you shift from condition Yellow (Relaxed But Aware) to condition Orange (Deliberately Aware).

You may make this harmless shift many times a day as you go about your normal routine. If someone or something looks out of place, you change from a 360-degree *general* awareness to a more *focused* concentration in a specific direction. At the same time, you can't drop your general awareness, because the threat in front of you may be a distraction for another behind.

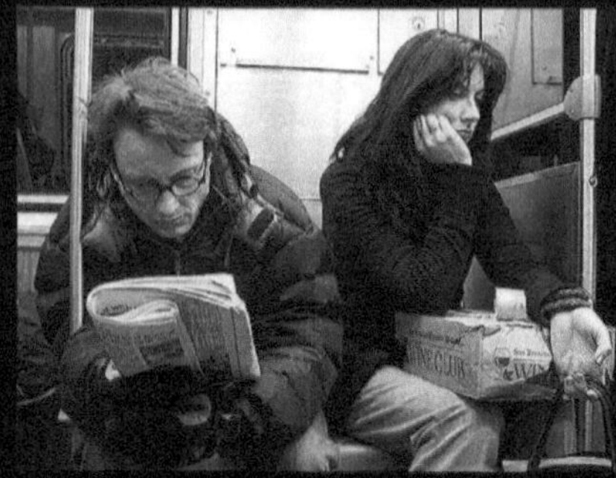

Condition WHITE

UNAWARE
and
OBLIVIOUS


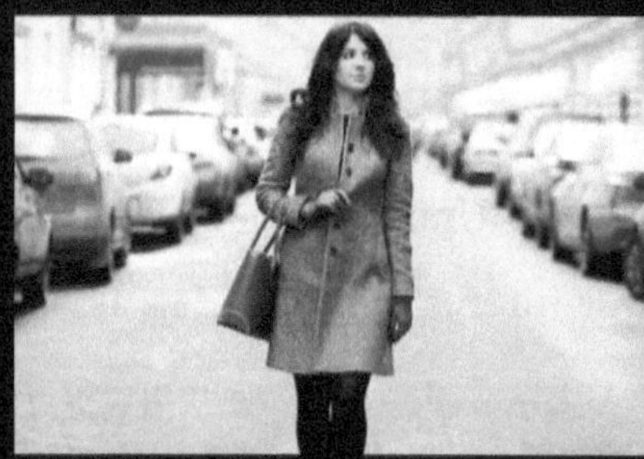

Condition YELLOW

RELAXED
but
AWARE


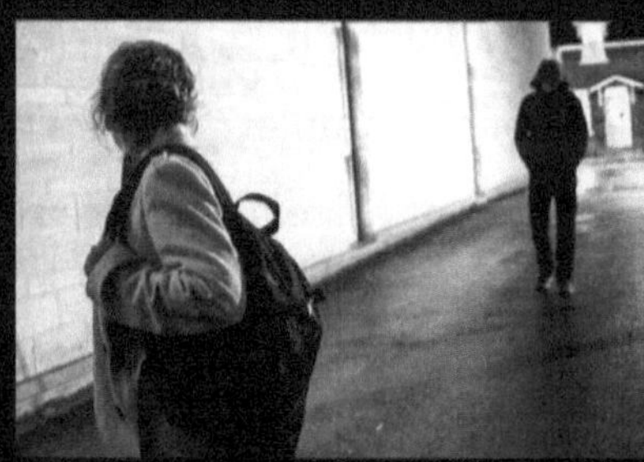

Condition ORANGE

ALERT
to a
POTENTIAL THREAT


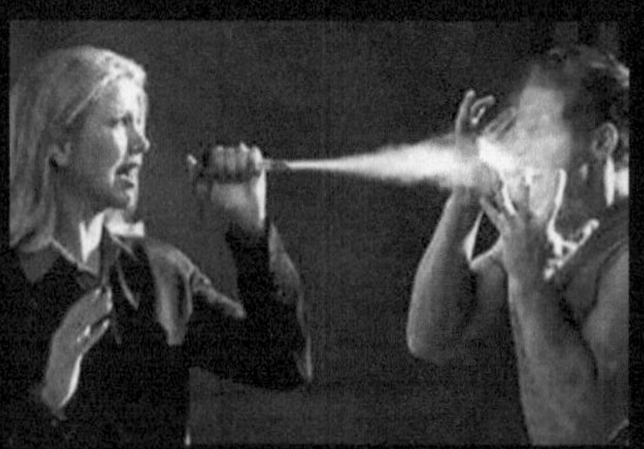

Condition RED

RESPOND
to the
ACTUAL THREAT

If you are attacked in condition Orange, you should be expecting the attack. Further, you will hopefully be facing your attacker since you have already shifted your focus in his direction. If you are well trained, your subconscious mind will have been considering possible response options based on past training sessions or similar events you have already experienced.

**Condition Red**

If the focus of your attention in condition Orange does something you find threatening, you will shift to condition Red. Note here that condition Red is not the combative engagement trigger, as some instructors have misconstrued from Cooper's teachings. Condition Red simply changes the focus of your attention from a potential **threat** to a potential **target**. You will physically respond, or take evasive action, only if the potential subject's actions dictate such a response.

Once you've shifted to condition Red, you cannot be surprised by your primary adversary and you are fully prepared to act decisively if the situation escalates further. Note, however, that your intense attention on a forward threat will lessen your ability to maintain 360-degree awareness for unknown threats that may come from other directions. Training under high-stress scenarios will help you avoid the *tunnel vision* that some describe as "looking through a tube of toilet paper."

If possible, in *both* conditions Orange and Red, move to a position that will give you a tactical advantage. Ideally, you want a wall or previously cleared area behind you, and some sort of solid cover you can move behind should violence erupt. Having one or more friends or acquaintances at this point can greatly enhance situational awareness, if—and only *if*—one of those friends remains alert in all directions; a rear guard, so to speak. Too often, everyone on the scene concentrates on the primary threat without maintaining the necessary 360-degree alertness.

If you are attacked in condition Red, you should be fully prepared to defend yourself **without reservation**. Whether or not you have an actual or improvised weapon on hand will depend on the circumstances—but mentally you must be already ahead of the game.

# HEARING WHAT IS NOT SAID

*An Alternative to Haragei*

Another set of ninjutsu teachings you should learn is *"Hearing What is Not Said."* This can be done by recognizing the four tactics used by predators when setting up their chosen targets for an attack. These tactics are sometimes referred to as the **Four Ds of Assailant Behavior**, and are especially popular with muggers and rapists. While these tactics are almost always overlooked by self-defense instructors, the Four D's—**Dialogue**, **Deception**, **Distraction**, and **Destruction** —are among the most important elements of self-protection to be aware of.

## Dialogue

Dialogue designed to disarm and distract the targeted individual is the professional attacker's most common priming technique. The attacker approaches a potential target in a non-threatening manner and initiates a conversation. Often, he will ask a question about directions, ask for the correct time, a light, or any spare change. This is what stage magicians call *misdirecion* and the attacker's objective is to preoccupy your mind with his question. You do not notice his encroaching proximity, his accomplice coming up behind you, or the weapon he is drawing. It only takes a second of distraction for your guard to drop, and for him to get past you defenses. Realizing this will keep you more alert, which is the most important part of target hardening.

**Target Hardening**

The term *target hardening* refers to the strengthening of security protection for an individual, a home, or a building in order to minimize the risk of a security-related breach. Target hardening includes measures and strategies designed to—

- keep an individual physically safe from all forms of threats
- ensure all residential and workplace facility doors and windows can resist forcible attacks, and
- physical barriers and landscapes can resist pedestrian intrusion.

## Deception

An attacker uses deception to make himself appear harmless. Dialogue and appearance are the most common methods used to deceive targets, to make them let down their guard. Do not expect dangerous people to stand out in a crowd.

Attacks may start with politeness, even with an ingratiating approach. Deception is the attacker's preferred tactic. Other than using a direct, blind-side attack, most street assaults rely on some ruse or pretext, with the attacker using this as a window of opportunity.

## Distraction

Distraction is a part of deception and usually comes through dialogue. The attacker may ask his target a question and then initiate attack while the target is thinking about the answer. This distraction typically switches off any instinctive, spontaneous physical response the target may have.

Brain engagement, whether by deceeptive or distracting dialogue, creates a momentary attention deficit in the target—which is all that is needed for the assailant to strike. The distraction is also used by the experienced attacker to redirect his target's mental status from one of caution and wariness to one of cooperation and, ideally for a predator, trust.

## Destruction

This is the final phase of an expert "set-up." Few people survive the first physical blow and most are out of the game before they even realize that they are in it. Even trained martial artists often get drawn in by the Four D's because these do not generally covered on their training curriculum; they do not understand the enemy they are facing. The attacker uses the techniques of deception and distraction to set up individuals who may be trained in recognize an overt threats but not an approach by deception.

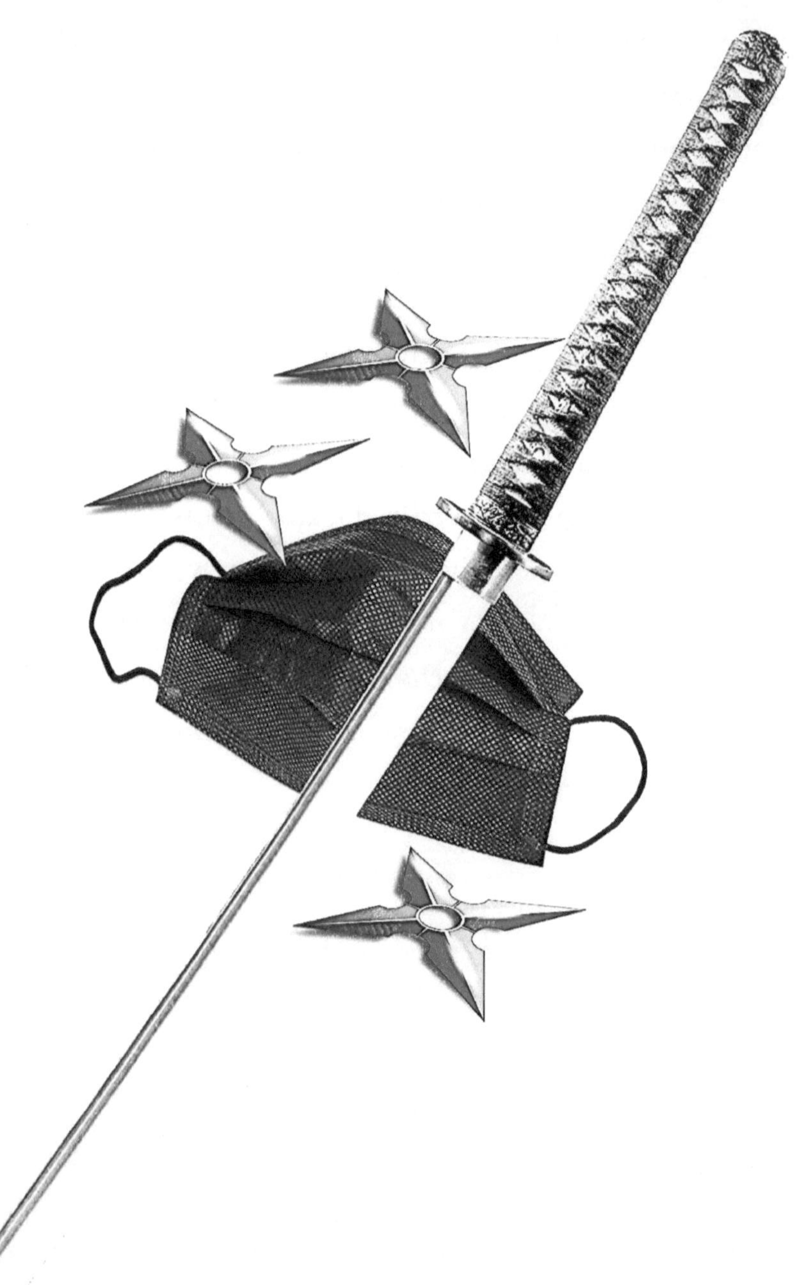

# SEEING WHAT IS NOT SHOWN



*An Alternative to Shinshin Shingan*

Another equally advanced set of teachings related to having the *Mind and Eyes of God*, is *Dokushin*, or "reading the enemy's intent." Like the many other talents attributed to them—scaling up castle wall, walking on water, turning into smoke, and disappearing like ghosts— *dokushin* was another "supernatural ability" based on the *shinobi*'s understanding and use of opponent psychology.

Though we all know we should be aware, very few self-protection programs specifically address *what* you should be aware of. The answer is: aware of **danger signs**, often known as pre-incident indicators, which are the specific actions that criminals or violent individuals perform in the moments immediately preceding an attack.

Knowing what these pre-incident indicators are and what they look like is one of the most important personal protection skills you can have. Even if you aren't able to avoid trouble completely, being aware of these pre-incident indicators will maximize your options in a critical situation and give you additional time to prepare and execute your response.

**Human Nature**

Violently attacking another person without warning is, for most, an unnatural act. That doesn't mean people aren't capable of it or that some don't do it quite regularly. It does mean that such an act is outside the normal realm of human behavior. And people who intend to act violently usually overcompensate in their attempts to appear normal beforehand. They also do things to set themselves up for success, which are obvious if you know what to look for. What follows are some of the most common pre-incident indicators and tips on how to recognize them more readily.

## Grooming

One of the most telling pre-incident indicators is what's known as *grooming*. People with malicious intent try very hard to look casual to avoid spooking their targets. Casual grooming actions like smoothing your hair with your fingers, scratching or wiping your face, or any similar unconscious gestures look very contrived and unnatural when done consciously. In simple terms, if you see someone trying *too* hard to look natural, *it's unnatural and a sign of potential danger.* Such behaviors very often precedes violent criminal attacks but can also signal the fact that a verbal altercation is about to become physical.

## Furtive Scanning

Criminals are always wary of potential witnesses. When sizing someone up as a target, a final action right *before* the attacks is to scan for witnesses. Again, the natural action of looking around appears a lot more suspicious when it's done purposefully. When it's done in conjunction with other pre-incident indicators, it's even more noticeable. For example, if you're walking near someone seated on a bench and he suddenly gets up, walks toward you and starts scanning the area as he approaches, warning bells should start going off in your head.

Such glances can also be in the form of unnatural eye movements. If normal individuals hear a noise or catch something out of the corner of their eyes, they will naturally turn their heads to look at the source of the stimulus. A person with ill intent, however, will often try to keep his head "naturally" pointing in one direction while looking to the sides for witnesses or to see if his intended target is paying attention. This Felix-the-Cat type of eye movement is unnatural and typically an indicator that the person is up to no good.

## Target Glancing

Before the assault, attackers will often pick a specific target to strike, visually focusing on it. If someone suddenly fixates on your chin, stomach or some other body part, he's probably not admiring your physique. Target glancing can also involve your personal belongings; if you notice someone staring at your jewelry, your laptop, or some other high-value possession, get your guard up and be ready to act

## Boundary Testing

Most criminals evaluate their targets before making the decision to attack. One of the most common ways of doing this is to engage the potential target with some type of question to test the person's boundaries and awareness. A classic example of this is asking for something like the time, change for a dollar and so forth. If your response is to look down at your watch or dig your hand in your pocket while allowing a stranger to move close to you, you're lowering your guard and allowing your boundaries to be violated. Don't let that happen to you!

## Coordinated Motion

Another potential cause for concern is someone coordinating their motion with yours. For example, if you're walking through a park and a seated person suddenly gets up to follow you, to walk parallel to you or to walk on a convergent course, that's suspicious. If two people begin moving simultaneously or seem to be coordinating their movement to trap you between them, that's an even bigger tell. Watch for others' unnatural reactions to your presence and be prepared to change the dynamics of the situation to keep yourself safe.

## Closing Distance

In Western society, we are used to maintaining a comfortable distance especially if there aren't many people around. For example, if you're on a subway platform full of empty benches and there's only one other person in sight, it would be unnatural for that person—a stranger—to try to sit down right next to you. Even if he decided to speak to you, he would typically do so from a respectable distance.

An attacker, however, wants to get close to you because attacks launched from close range give you less time to react. This may be done by simply walking up to you, by sitting next to you or through a more subtle means known as boundary testing.

## Hiding the Hands

When people walk naturally, they swing their arms and their hands are open. A person hiding a weapon, however, may move very differently. If the weapon is concealed behind his leg or back, that arm will not swing naturally as he walks. If a small weapon like a knife is hidden in the hand, the fingers will not be naturally extended or the thumb may not be visible. Similarly, a person preparing to attack with a punch may unconsciously clench his fists well before he begins swinging. If you don't see naturally extended fingers and a normal arm swing, be prepared.

Hidden hands may also mean the hands are concealed in pockets. A person approaching you with his hands in his pockets or jacket may be preparing to draw a weapon. Shouting the simple phrase *"Show me your hands!"* at the person and from a safe reactive distance can be a game changer. Also make note of people *openly* carrying ordinary objects in their hands that could be used as improvised weapons—especially things like bottles.

## Weight Shifting

One very disturbing form of violent crime that has become popular in recent years is the *Knockout Game,* the goal being to knock out an unsuspecting target in public with a single punch. This approach is also common with robbers who approach their targets and, without warning, knock them down with a haymaker punch before stealing their valuables.

For most people, delivering a knockout punch requires *a wind up.* Typically this is a rearward shift of body weight and a bending of the back leg to create both rotation and drive to power the punch. In many cases, the rear shoulder will drop and the attacker will actually look away before turning back to the target to strike. Weight shifting is often preceded or combined with other indicators like **target glancing**, **scanning for witnesses** and **grooming** actions. As obvious as these actions may seem, most people respond like the *deer in the headlights*—and they do nothing to react.

# Part IV:

# Staying Honed

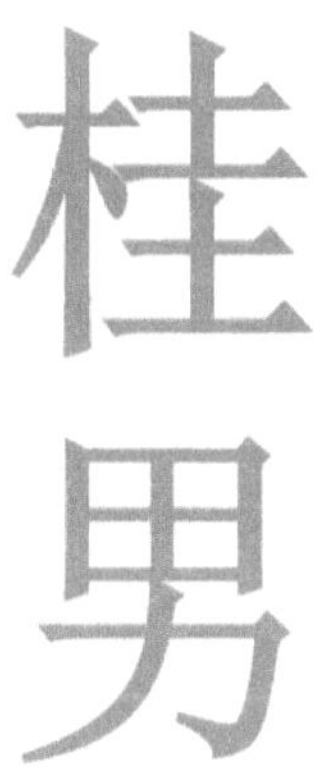

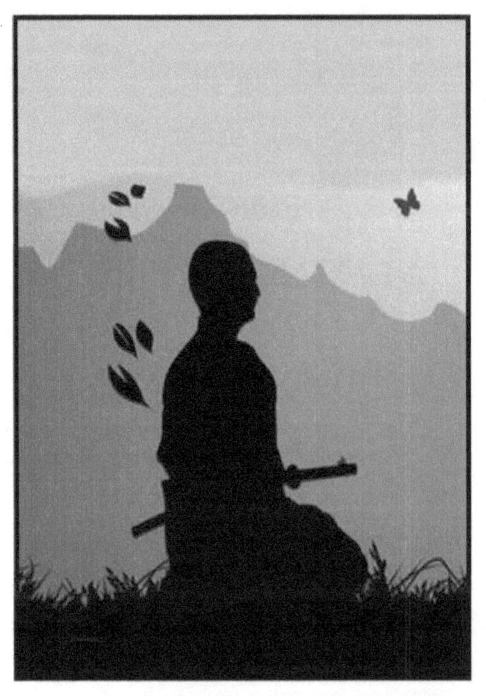

When a person experiences certain emotions—fear, for example—their reflex and non-conscious response of holding their breath elevates tension on both the physical and mental levels. It can also happen with extreme feelings of surprise, grief, joy, and anger, to list the more common ones.

It can happen the other way as well; we can non-consciously alter breathing to avoid feeling an undesired emotion. This is because we know that breathing can generate and fuel emotion. If a child dreads feeling sadness, anger, or fear, he may stifle his breath to avoid crying or feeling something uncomfortable. As adults we may still inhibit our breathing to keep unwanted feelings repressed.

### Inadequate Patterns of Breathing

Inadequate patterns of breathing also lead to anxiety, irritability, and tension. Such symptoms are the basis for claustrophobia, agoraphobia, and other anxiety disorders. Claustrophobic people feel they are unable to get enough air in closed spaces, while agoraphobics are afraid of open spaces because the outdoors stimulate their breathing. Any breathing difficulty will create anxiety, and when this difficulty is severe it leads to panic, fear, and potentially terror.

During times of emotional stress our sympathetic nervous system is stimulated and effects a number of physical responses. Our heart rate rises, we perspire, our muscles tense, and our breathing becomes rapid and shallow. If this process happens over a long period of time, the sympathetic nervous system becomes over-stimulated, leading to an imbalance that can affect our physical health and result in inflammation, high blood pressure, and muscle pain to name a few.

Fortunately, by becoming aware of how we breathe, we can *consciously*[10] regain control of our respiration and take an active role over our tensions, fears, and other extreme emotions.

## Strengthening the Mind-Body Connection

Breathing is the essence of being, and *conscious breathing* is a process that is well understood by many Asian cultures. A rhythmic *cycle* of expansion and contraction, breathing is one example of the consistent polarity we see in nature such as night and day, wake and sleep, seasonal growth and decay, and ultimately life and death.

Breathing is the only bodily function that we do both voluntarily and involuntarily. Unlike the other bodily functions, the breath is easily used to communicate between these systems, and can be an excellent tool to help facilitate positive change. Although some might think that consciously attempting to slow our heart rate, decrease perspiration, or relax our muscles is an extremely difficult task unless we have undertaken long and arduous ascetic training of *yamabushi* and *shugenya* warriors, we can easily use breathing to consciously influence the involuntary (sympathetic nervous system) that regulates

_______________

10 As opposed to the *non-conscious* and unintended behaviors already discussed.

blood pressure, heart rate, circulation, digestion, and many other bodily functions.

Proper breathing techniques act as a bridge into those functions of the body over which we generally do not have conscious control. (We know how our bodies know to do this naturally when we take a deep breath or sigh when a stress is relieved.) Learning and using proper breathing techniques is one of the most beneficial disciplines a ninjutsu exponent can practice to direct his short- and long-term physical and emotional health.

### The Benefits of *Fukushiki Kokyu*

The *koryū bugei* practice of *fukushiki kokyu*, which is widely-used in many of the combat arts, also serves as a fundamental means for the development of *shinrigaku* disciplines. It is of particular and proven value in the enhancement of the haragei and kiaijutsu abilities already discussed.

The practice of *fukushiki kokyu* is similar to what is known today as abdominal or diaphragmatic breathing. The diaphragm, as we already know, is the large muscle located between the chest and the abdomen. When it contracts it is forced downward causing the abdomen to expand. This causes a negative pressure within the chest forcing air into the lungs.

The negative pressure also pulls blood into the chest improving the venous return to the heart. This leads to improved stamina in both athletic activity and disease. Like blood, the flow of lymph, which is rich in immune cells, is also improved. By expanding the lung's air pockets and improving the flow of blood and lymph, *fukushiki kokyu* breathing also helps prevent infection of the lung and other tissues.

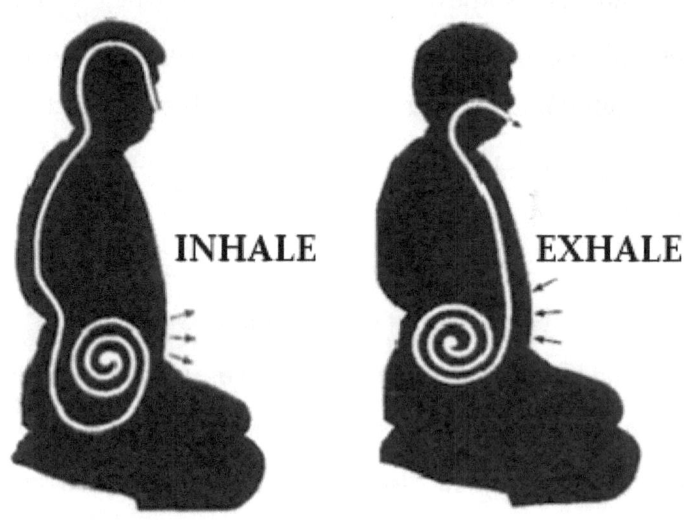


### Levels of Fukushiki Kokyu Training

*Fukushiki kokyu* breathing exercises should be practiced twice a day, as well as when your mind is dwelling on upsetting thoughts, or when you are experiencing pain. The easiest regimen is to practice when you wake every morning and in the evening when you retire. Each session takes only about three minutes to complete. When one neglects to make the minimal time and effort needed to practice these simple exercises, he is not merely a forfeiting a known benefit, but actually stagnating and sabotaging his ninjutsu abilities and development.

**Beginner Level Training**

In the initial *learning* stage of your training:

1. Lie down on your tatami, and consciously release all innate muscular tension

2. Place one hand on your chest and the other on your abdomen. The hand on your chest will confirm that it does *not* rise or expand, while the hand on your abdomen will confirm that it rises and "inflates." This will also ensures that the diaphragm is pulling air into the bases of the lungs

3. Press your tongue under your palate and just behind your upper teeth

4. To begin, inhale a slow deep breath *through your nose* imagining that you are pulling in all the air in the room into your *hara* for a *steady count of 4*.

5. Hold your breath in the *hara*—without unnecessary tension— for a *steady count of 7*.

6. Relax your abdomen and slowly exhale *through your mouth* for *a count of 8*.

7. When all the air is released, *gently*[11] contract your abdominal muscles to completely evacuate any remaining air from the lower lungs. *It is important to note that we deepen respiration not by inhaling more air but by completely exhaling it.*

8. Repeat the *fukushiki kokyu* breathing cycle seven more times for a total of eight (8) deep repetitions.

---

11 Avoid doing this forcefully, as some instructors teach, because this can create a counter-productive muscular tension

## Middle Level Training

Once you are familiar and adept with the above technique while lying down, you should begin to practice it while sitting—relaxed[12]—in a chair. At this stage of training you should no longer need to use your hands to monitor chest and abdomen movement. Instead, place your hands, in a reverse clasped manner, on your legs and below the *hara*.

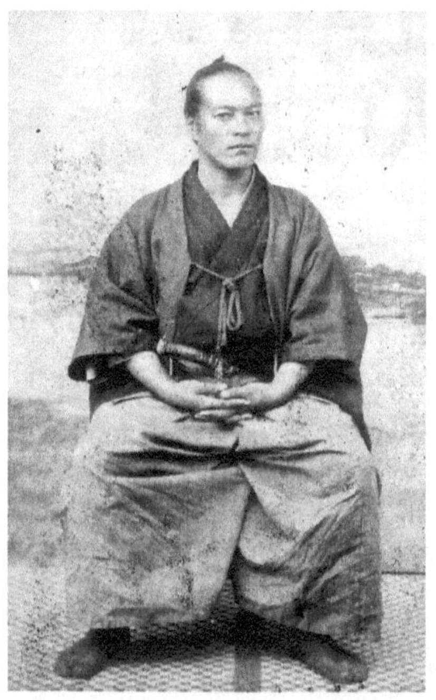

Yamaoka Tesshu seated in the manner described

After you are successful in sitting *fukushiki kokyu* practice you should, when ready, advance to practice from a *seiza* position. However, you will only be ready if sitting in *seiza* for the duration of the eight repetitions does not cause physical distress, or if your discomfort does not become a distraction.

---

12 But not slouched.

74

**Advanced Level Training**

The *Shoden* (beginner teachings) and *Chuden* (middle teachings) levels of *fukushiki kokyu* practice are related to the *Katsusatsu* healing disciplines of ninjutsu. At the *Okuden* (advanced teachings) level, *fukushiki kokyu* practice moves into the realm of *Shinrigaku* mental disciplines.

At this *Okuden* level, you add directed and deliberate *emotional* content to your practice. This level of *fukushiki kokyu* practice may be performed while sitting in a chair or in *seiza*. The practice involves incorporating **specific words** that enhance the results of the exercise.

The specific words you choose to incorporate into your breathing will always be in *matched pairs*. The first word of the pair will describe a *personal quality* you are summoning or confirming; the second word will describe a *negative feeling or emotion* that you are rejecting or eliminating. This is not as challenging or confusing as it may sound. Examples of matched pairs of words would be:

> ***relaxed – anger***, or
>
> ***confident – fear***

Thus, as you engage in *fukushiki kokyu* practice,

- mentally "say" the word "relaxed" along with your 4-count inhalation
- hold the thought of that personal quality, of being *relaxed*, for your 7-count, then

- reject and expel the negative emotion or feeling, in this case *anger*, during your exhalation.

The intent is simply to *summon* the personal quality you want with the inhalation and *dispel* any negative feelings with the exhalation. When practicing *fukushiki kokyu* at the Okuden level, the *exhalation* should be *three* times as long as inhalation; that is, for *a steady count to 12*. So, inhale for 4; hold for 7; *exhale for 12*.

# SEALING THE GAPS IN YOUR ARMOR

It is a fact not well known that in time of war the shinobi, like the samurai, could also opt to wear *kusari katabira yoroi*; that is, a light-weight armor (*yoroi*) made of chain mail. This happened infrequently, however, because the shinobi valued mobility, agility, and quiet movement—all of which were compromised by wearing yoroi.

The light armor was intended to provide a modicum of protection in open battle, but even when wearing it the ninja was not entirely immune to an enemy's attacks. This was because every known type of armor, whether European or Asian in origin, contains gaps or weak points in their construction—dangerous gaps that allow penetration by a skilled enemy wielding a sharp-pointed weapon.

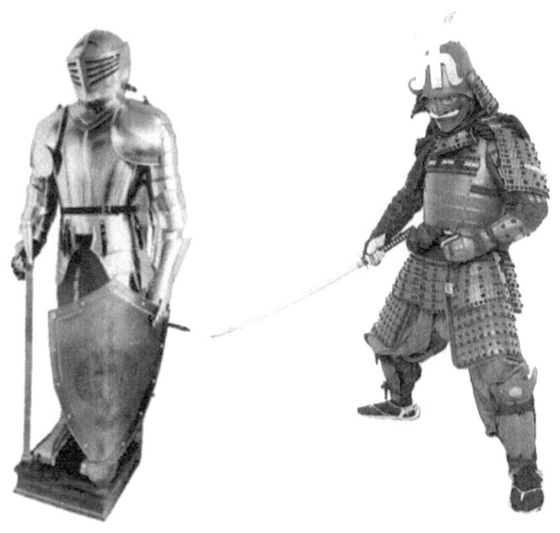

**Every known type of armor contains gaps or weak points**

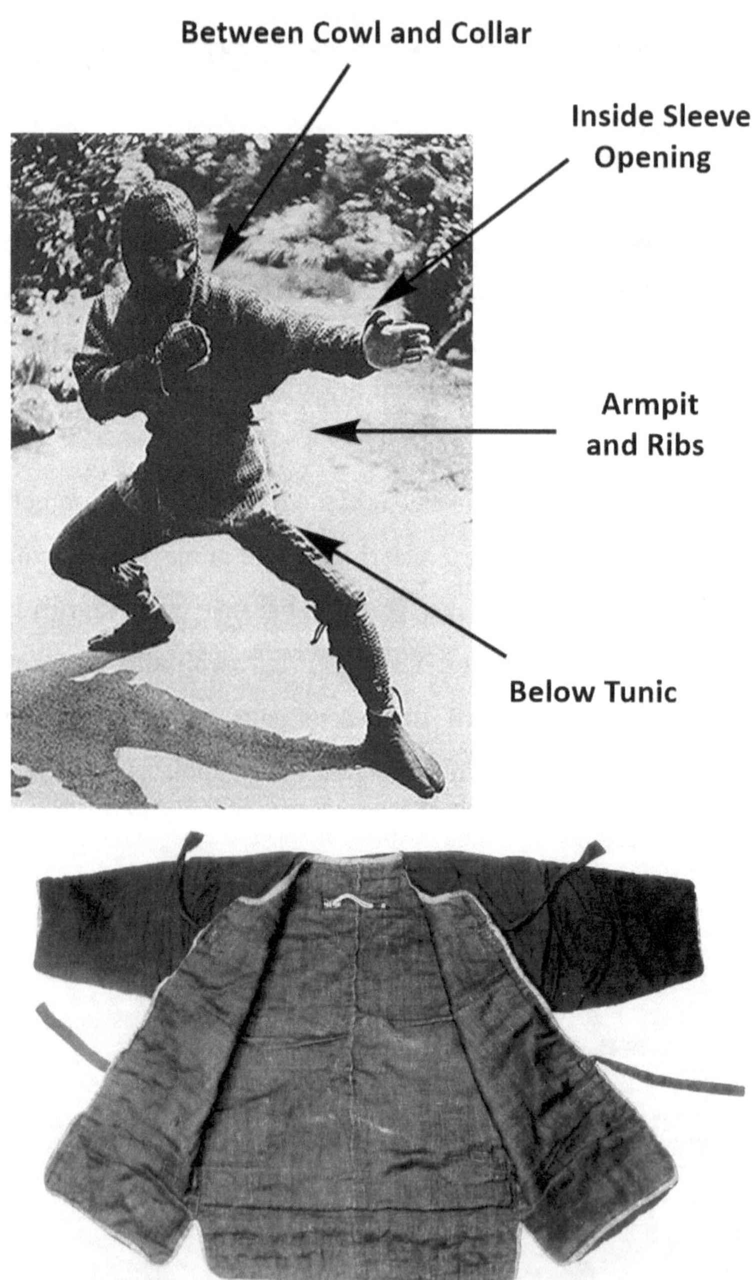



*Above,* **A ninja in light chain mail armor**
*Below,* **open view of top section**

**The Yoroi Analogy**

The gaps are called *chinks* in western armor and *suki* in Japanese. As a consequence of this vulnerability, both the shinobi and the samurai had to remain mindful of their *suki* even when they thought themselves protected. You may currently be taking the proper precautions—frequent hand-washing, using hand sanitizer, wearing an appropriate mask, and maintaining social distance—intending that to be your "armor." But the parallel is clear: you too must be mindful of potential gaps in your precautions *even when you think yourself protected.*

**Mind Your** (Potential) **Gaps**

The *suki* in your *yoroi*, or gaps in your armor, are the potential bad habits that can develop from yearning for your former normalcy. You may become tired, or lazy, or bored with your mundane safety procedures, or become brazen and overconfident from being healthy and unaffected. You are conveniently forgetting that it is the safety procedures you have followed that have kept you that way.

Below is a short list of the potential gaps that can threaten the armor of your diligent practices—

Suki 1. **Gradual Lessening of Safeguard Disciplines**

> Fear of the unknown is a common driver for people to take action. In the early days of the pandemic, when little was known about the virus, its mysteriousness prompted people to take protective measures seriously. However, familiarity breeds contempt and living with the threat of the virus over the span

of time can normalize it and make people more lax about maintaining their discipline.

The key to avoiding this mistake is to act as if you are just learning about the virus. "Repeated creative reminders linked to the evolving situation are important to avoid complacency," says one study.

### Suki 2. **Diregarding Everyday Hazards**

The pandemic crisis has our attention right now, so we are hyper-focused on mitigating the risk of exposure to it. But over-focusing on one potential hazard may cause some to neglect *other* everyday basics that keep them healthy. Ongoing sleep, regular exercise, and human companionship all require continued attention, which is contrary to an overwhelming attitude that *all else can wait*.

### Suki 3. **Becoming Impatient for the Return to Normalcy**

Do you miss not being able to go to your dojo, or salle, or gym or getting together with friends on Friday nights? Of course, and that's normal. Human behavior is driven by a strong aversion to losses and a desire to maintain the status quo. But that desire for the status quo can be so strong that people dismiss the rules altogether. We must emphasize for ourselves our future gains to help us see past the status quo and understand the benefit of social distancing and the other related and required measures.

Suki 4. **Acting on Reflex Instead of Remaining Mindful**

Simple things like hugging a friend you run into at the grocery store or standing close to your neighbor when you're both out walking your dogs are habits that are hard to break. Human behavior is heavily influenced by deeply ingrained societal norms and when we have to abandon or change them, it can be difficult for people to follow through. You must stay informed, do your best, and if you forget, move forward without becoming obsessively upset about such changes.

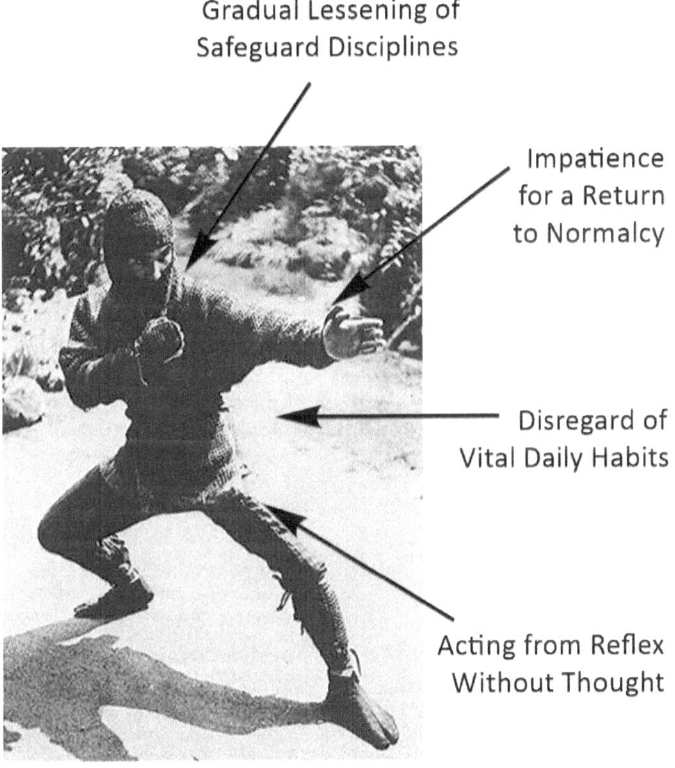


**The gaps in your armor are the potential bad habits that can develop over time. Always remember that it is the safeguards you have followed that have kept you healthy.**

Monitor these and other potential gaps in your armor. Staying on top of social distancing—and all the other precautions—for months on end—isn't easy, and the  new normal will require being extra conscious of the pitfalls on this list. But it's worth remembering that we won't have to live this way forever. Temporary measures will lead to longer lasting safety.

# CLOSING THOUGHTS

The insidious danger posed by the current pandemic is different from the type of threats you typically face from opponents in the dojo, the fencing salle, the boxing gym, or the firearms range. The differences are many and obvious; for example—

- an opponent's approach can usually be observed; yet such is not the case with an infectious agent which, like a vicious knife thrust, is felt but rarely seen.

- an opponent is found in a dojo, a salle, a gym, a dark street, and places you might expect; but not an infectious agent, which can be present in the most innocuous-looking person and in the most harmless-seeming venue.

- an opponent attacks within a known set of parameters; but not an infectious agent, which follows no predictable protocols prior to attacking.

In essence, you cannot defend against disease by the skillful use of punches or kicks, chokes, locks, or throws, or even of a saber or a handgun. Therefore, as is true of all threats, prevention is your best defense, and one always preferable to requiring a cure.

## Physical Skills and Mental Attributes

Fortunately, as an individual who trains in defensive techniques and tactics, you already possess a great number of physical skills and mental attributes that can optimize your prevention strategies and enhance the safeguards you already follow. Formally-structured

Eastern or Western combat disciplines provide you with a unique assortment of abilities and sensibilities that can reliably serve you beyond the walls of your training hall. Drawing from the many tenets commonly taught in most fighting arts, you can utilize the  attributes you have learned to minimize potential exposure to infection in the same way you have learned to avoid potential assailants.

**Three-Layered Defense Strategy**

Thinking of an infectious disease as an "attacker" will help you establish a workable defense strategy. Begin by realizing that, generally speaking:

- **proximity** or **approach** by unknown others is your primary danger;
- **limiting** or **denying proximity**—and maintaining a safe distance—is your principal defense against that danger.

The strategy for denying of proximity and the maintenance of a safe distance is comprised of three tactics: 1) *Avoiding*, 2) *Evading*, and 3) *Intervening*.

### Avoid

The first tactic in your defense is avoidance, and depends on the proper use of your eyes to:

—routinely *scan* your immediate environment when in the company of others

—*identify* anyone unknown to you who appears to be approaching too close

—use your gaze to *communicate* your concern to anyone encroaching on safety zone. The proper use of the gaze is covered in the chapter on *Metsuke* (*page 35.*)

## Evade

If avoiding them is not an option, a second tactic for denying proximity is evasion. Use footwork that is somewhat reminiscent to how you walk or stand when someone starts to come inordinateky close to you at a social function. This concept is known as *musubi* in Japanese, and simply refers to the way we non-consciously but fuidly avoid colliding with people in crowded malls, theaters, and airports.

## Intervene

On the rare occasion when neither avoidance or evasion are workable responses, your third and final tactic will be intervention. In this sense, intervention refers to a respectful but assertive reminder to another to not approach any closer. This *reminder* can be non-verbally communicated by, again respectfully, extending your palm toward them to stop their approach. Alternatively it can take the form of telling them to keep their distance. *"Excuse me! Six feet away please ..."* Always be mindful that whether you express your reminder non-verbally or verbally, the tone you employ will greatly influence how your message is received.

*Please Stay Safe;*
*and whether you do so in a health-minded group or by yourself*
*keep on training!*

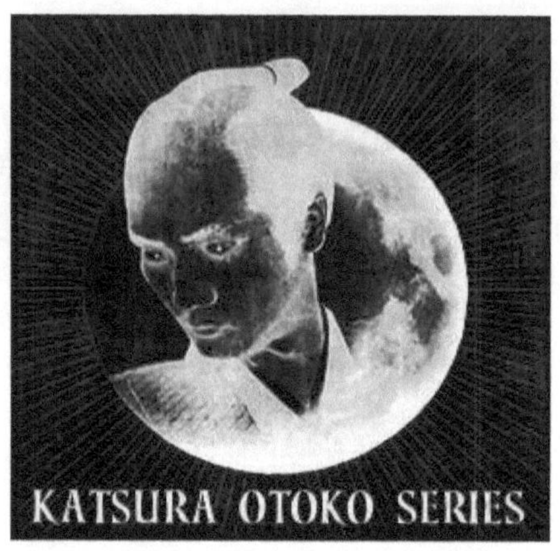


The shinobi existing under constant threat
lives his/her life removed from the dangers around him,
like *katsura otoko*—the Man on the Moon.

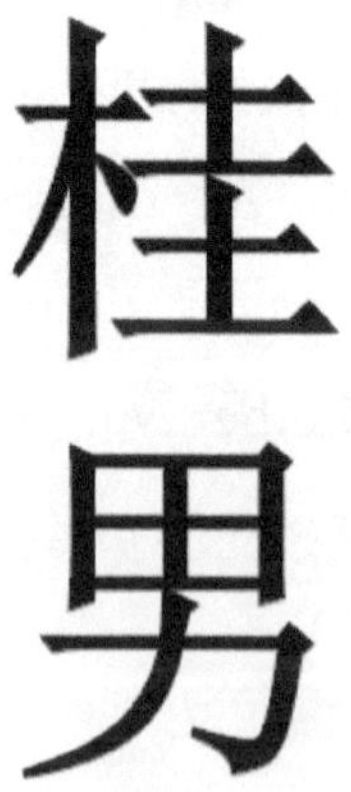

# GLOSSARY

Below is a glossary of the more unfamiliar terms used throughout this volume. The glossary does not include every Japanese term, nor are the definitions provided meant to be comprehensive or definitive in scope.

**Banpen Fugyo**    "Ten Thousand Changes, No Surprises" The mental attitude that one will not become flustered or emotionally altered by unexpected changes.

**Bushi**    "Military person or warrior"; a samurai

**Bugei**    "Military craft"; traditional fighting arts developed and practiced prior to 1868, after which samurai were mandated to give up the sword.

**Fukushiki Kokyu**    A common form of diaphragmatic breathing used to enhance martial awareness and sensitivity to danger

**Gendai Budo**    "Modern Martial Ways" Fighting arts originating after 1868, i.e., *Aikido, Judo, Karate, etc.* See also *Koryu Bugei*

**Haragei**    "Stomach art" A finely-developed "gut feeling" that allows one to perceive another person's true but concealed intentions

**Heiho**    "Military strategy"

**IMINT**    Intelligence community acronym for *Imagery Intelligence*, referring to information gathered via aerial photography and similar means

**Koryu Bugei**    "Ancient Martial Arts" Traditional fighting arts developed and used prior to 1868 and actually used in war, e,g. *Kenjutsu, Kyujutsu, Ninjutsu,* etc. See also *Gendai Budo*

**Katsura Otoko**    "The Man on the Moon" A long-term strategy for an active ninja to live alone, without support, behind enemy lines

| | |
|---|---|
| **Ninja** | Modern term for a specialist in **Ninjutsu**, the Japanese art of *Intelligence-Gathering and Espionage*. See also, *Shinobi* |
| **Ninjutsu** | The Japanese art of Intelligence-Gathering and Espionage, more properly called **shinobijutsu**, *first codified in the 15th century.* |
| **OSINT** | Intelligence community acronym for *Open Source Intelligence*, referring to information gathered from publicly available (non-proprietary) documents |
| **Pre-Incident Indicator** | A behavioral cue of an assailant's intent to attack. There are many such cues that are inadvertently "leaked" by the assailant and can be read *in advance* |
| **Samurai** | "One who serves" Similar to the Western notion of a knight, the *samurai* or *bushi* was an elite fighting man in service to a lord. |
| **Shinobi** | Proper name for *ninja,* a practitioner of the art of *Ninjutsu.* A specialist in espionage and covert activities |
| **Shinobijutsu** | Proper name for ninjutsu, the *Art of Espionage and Subterfuge* |
| **Shinrigaku** | "Martial Psychology" Mental and psychological techniques and tactics designed to defeat an enemy |
| **Shinshin Shingan** | "The Mind and Eyes of God" A martial attribute that allows one to foresee or pre-sense the danger in a situation |
| **SIGINT** | Intelligence community acronym for *Signals Intelligence*, referring to information gathered from intercepted electronic communications via satellites and other forms of eavesdropping |
| **Sonbu** | Japanese name for *Sun Tzu,* the presumed author of *The Art of War* |
| **Sonshi** | Japanese name for the Chinese treatise known as *The Art of War* |
| **Suki** | A vulnerable gap in armor |
| **Sun Tzu** | One of various Chinese names ascribed to a warrior-philosopher who is belied to have written the *Bing Fa, The Art of War* |
| **Yoroi** | Japanese Armor |

# ABOUT THE AUTHOR

In 1984, James Loriega founded the **New York Ninpokai**, a training facility which came to be regarded as *"the premier academy for the traditional shinobi arts in NYC."* Loriega began his formal martial arts training in 1967 with the late Grandmaster Ronald Duncan, the first non-Japanese to teach the shinobi arts in the United States—and the acknowledged *Father of American Ninjutsu.* Though he later trained with other ninjutsu masters, it was from Duncan-sensei that Loriega learned the myriad strategies, tactics, techniques, and disciplines of the ancient *shinobi.*

During the mid- to late-80s, Loriega also studied other Japanese martial arts, including *Aikijujutsu, Taijutsu, Jojutsu, and Hojojutsu.* Loriega began writing extensively around that same time, and from 1985 to 1995 served as Technical Consultant and Contributing Editor for **Ninja** magazine, an international publication dedicated exclusively to ninjutsu.

In February of 2018, he was recognized by the *Martial Arts University* as a *Martial Arts Icon*—an individual who is symbolic of an idea and leaves a memorable mark on the lives of those he teaches.

In April of 2018, he was recognized as a *Ninjutsu Scholar* and inducted into the *International Circle of Masters* (ICM).

Loriega holds instructor ranks in Ninjutsu, Jujutsu, and Aikijujutsu, as well as in a number of Western martial arts. He has published over a thirty books on martial arts, martial culture, and espionage tradecraft, and his extensive writings have appeared in mainstream martial arts publications such as **Black Belt**, **Inside Kung-Fu**, **Ninja**, and **Tactical Knives**.

*Inquiries for seminars or workshops may be sent to:*

Ninpokai@aol.com

# BIBLIOGRAPHY

Adams, Andrew. **Ninja**, *The Invisible Assassins*. Burbank, Ca: Ohara Publication. 1971

Cummins, Antony. **Iga and Koka Ninja Skills**: *The Secret Shinobi Scrolls of Chikamatsu Shigenori*. Gloucestershire, UK: The History Press. 2013

deBecker, Gavin. **The Gift of Fear**. New York: Little, Brown and Company. 1997

Draeger, Donn F. and Robert W. Smith. **Asian Fighting Arts**. Tokyo, New York, San Francisco: Kodansha International, Ltd. 1969

– **Ninjutsu,** *The Art of Invisibility.* Tokyo: Lotus Press. 1971

– **Classical Bujutsu**. New York: John Weatherhill, Inc. 1973

Gilbey, John. (Pen name for Robert W. Smith) **Secret Fighting Arts of the World**. Rutland, Vt. and Tokyo, Japan: Charles E. Tuttle Co. 1963

Gluck, Jay, **Zen Combat**. New York: Ballantine Books. 1962

Harrison, E. J. **The Fighting Spirit of Japan.** London: Unwin. 1912

Hayes, Stephen K. **The Ninja and Their Secret Fighting Art**. Rutland, VT and Tokyo, Japan: Charles E. Tuttle Co. 1981

Hirose, Junzo. **Unknown Ninja**: *Shinobi Agents in World War II.* New York: Lost Arts Publications. 2017

Loriega, James. **Ninso:** *Ninjutsu's Art of Face Reading*. New York: Pay-Per-Cut Press. 2017

– **Shinobi-no-Michi:** *A Legacy of Lost Arts*. New York: Lost Arts Publications. 2018

– **Katsura Otoko**: *Ninjutsu Training for the Lone Practitioner.* New York: Lost Arts Publications. 2018

– **The Divine Threads:** *An Origin of Ninjutsu*. New York: Lost Arts Publications. 2019

– **The Lost Writings of Ninjutsu**. New York: Lost Arts Publications. 2019

– **Life Strategies of a Master Spy:** *Advice from the First CIA Director***.** Washington, DC: Raven Tradecraft Press. 2019

– **Zankanjo**: *The Code of Shinobi*. New York: Lost Arts Publications. 2020

– **Shinobi Aruki**: *Walking Methods of the Modern Ninja*. New York: Lost Arts Publications. 2021

Musashi, Miyamoto. **The Book of Five Rings**. Thomas Cleary, translator. Boston: Shambala Books. 1993

Okuse, Heichishiro. **Ninjutsu Hiden** (忍術秘伝). Osaka, Japan: Bonbonsha. 1959

Onoda, Hiroo. **No Surrender:** *My Thirty Year War*. Charles S. Terry, translator. Tokyo, New York & San Francisco: Kodansha International. 1974

Seiko, Fujita. **What Is Ninjutsu?** Eric Shahan, translator. CreateSpace Independent Publishing. 2017

– **The Eighteen Weapons of War**. Eric Shahan, translator. CreateSpace Independent Publishing. 2017

Sun Tzu. **The Art of War.** Lionel Giles, translator. London: Lozac. 1910

Suzuki, Shunryu. **Zen Mind, Beginner's Mind**. New York: Weatherhill, Inc. 1970

Yagyu Munenori. **The Sword and the Mind**. Hiraoki Sato, translator. New York: The Overlook Press. 1986